YOU and HIV

A DAY AT A TIME

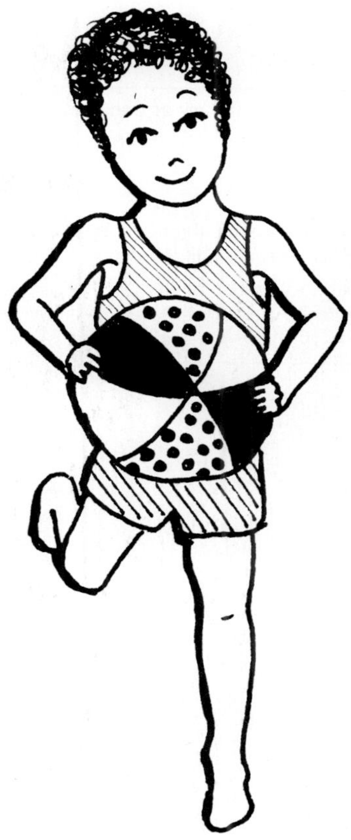

written and illustrated by

LYNN S. BAKER, M.D.

W.B. SAUNDERS COMPANY
Harcourt Brace Jovanovich, Inc.
Philadelphia London Toronto Montreal Sydney Tokyo

W. B. SAUNDERS COMPANY
Harcourt Brace Jovanovich, Inc.

The Curtis Center
Independence Square West
Philadelphia, PA 19106

Library of Congress Cataloging-in-Publication Data

Baker, Lynn S.
You and HIV : a day at a time / written and illustrated by Lynn S. Baker.
p. cm.
Includes bibliographical references and index.
1. AIDS (Disease) in children—Juvenile literature. I. Title.
RJ387. A25B35 1991
362.1'9892697'92—dc20 91-2802
ISBN 0-7216-3606-3

Editor: John Dyson

YOU AND HIV... A DAY AT A TIME ISBN 0-7216-3606-3

Printed in the United States of America

Last digit is the print number 9 8 7 6 5 4 3 2 1

Dedicated to

Aaron
Annalisa
Anthony
Ariel
Bouboute
Faith
Hydeia
Jeremy
Jessie
Joey
Josh
Keisha
Kiley
Kweisi
Melissa
Mikey
Patrick
Qiyam
Samuel
Tania
Zack
Zagia

to their families
and to you.

CONTENTS

PREFACE

In the mid-1970s, Lynn Baker published *You and Leukemia*. As a practicing pediatric oncologist, I found this book to be of incredible value. Written in a simple, clear manner, it provided an extraordinary array of information to children and parents about cancer—its causes, symptoms, treatments and complications. Even more important, it gave a voice and expression to the feelings and emotions of children experiencing a life-threatening illness. Such insights proved invaluable not only to patients and their families but also to their caregivers. I certainly benefited from reading *You and Leukemia*, since it offered a perspective on disease that was not available from medical texts or journals. In fact, I have always believed that *You and Leukemia* should be considered required reading for all who participate in the care of children with cancer.

Now, in the 1990s, Lynn Baker has produced *You and HIV*. Once again, Dr. Baker has addressed one of the most serious threats to the health of children and has provided an extraordinarily rich compendium of facts, feelings and issues. Although addressed to patients and parents, *You and HIV* will prove highly readable and informative to a wide audience. Indeed, students, social workers, teachers, health administrators, policy makers and virtually anyone interested in children with HIV infection would find this volume to be an exceptional primer. In my opinion, it comprises the simplest and most informative introduction to understanding the immune system and HIV that I have yet encountered. Moreover, the clinical manifestations of HIV infection and its treatment are covered in helpful and understandable detail. Even though the content of this volume will nearly always be above the level of the children who are infected, it should prove useful to virtually everyone involved in their care and treatment. Indeed, I would hope that everyone interested in children with HIV infection will read and learn from this most informative book.

PHILIP A. PIZZO, M.D.
Chief, Pediatric Branch
Head, Infectious Disease Section
National Cancer Institute
Professor of Pediatrics
Uniformed Services University
of the Health Sciences

FOREWORD

Understanding HIV and having the support of family and friends are the keys to "living with HIV." Dr. Lynn Baker has given children infected with the AIDS virus both that understanding and support.

Dr. Baker spent countless hours with families, understanding how HIV absorbs their lives. She listened as children, Moms and Dads vented their frustrations with this disease. She sensed their intense feelings of fear, inadequacy, and sometimes guilt, should their secret be discovered. She realized the need of those affected by HIV to live with dignity and to be given respect as human beings.

Dr. Baker's book, *You and HIV... A Day at a Time,* is an incredible resource guide for children with HIV infection and their families. It's an in-depth, cleverly illustrated work that details every aspect of this intricate disease. It enables the child to first understand a great deal about his own body and then clearly maps out the momentum of HIV infection.

The book is designed for parents and children, and devouring its content is a team effort. It assures support as it emphasizes how special the HIV-infected child is. Dr. Baker's book is an excellent resource guide for every physician's office. It carefully explains and examines procedures and treatments often encountered with this disease.

Disclosure of HIV infection to others is a decision each individual must make, and Dr. Baker gives us the knowledge to make that decision. Through *You and HIV... A Day at a Time,* she gives our kids the courage to "live with HIV." With her help, HIV will one day be a disease we can talk about openly and accurately.

DIANA J. DOWLING, *Parent*

INTRODUCTION

When I was three and four years old, I was very sick. I spent those years going in and out of the hospital and having all sorts of things done to my body, including an operation. One time I almost died from an allergic reaction to penicillin, but I didn't know it then. Even if I had known, I wouldn't have cared. I was concerned with living. To me, the worst thing that happened during that time was when my roommate, Julie, decided she hated me, would never speak to me again—and changed *her* name to "Audrey" because my *doll's* name was Julie. When you're little, things like that—rejection, separation, and loneliness—are much bigger deals than mortality.

I was also scared a lot, never knowing what was going to happen next, or why—or if it would hurt. I know how much it would have helped if someone had figured out that being little and being stupid were not the same thing, that I was capable of understanding and wanted to understand what was going on. By keeping me ignorant, those who loved and cared for me never gave me the chance to participate positively in my own illness—in my own *life.*

This book was written to give that chance to children with HIV and to help the people who care for and about them learn enough to be able to answer the endless questions curious children ask. It's a long book because HIV is a complicated illness and I wanted to take the time and the space to make HIV understandable to everyone.

Most books are meant to be read from beginning to end. This book is no different. The reason is that there are many words and ideas that you will need to be familiar with in order to understand HIV and its treatment. The first part of the book contains explanations of these words and ideas, and if you read this part first, the later sections should not be confusing.

In case you just want to read about certain subjects, I've done two things. The first is a comprehensive Index at the very back of the book that gives you the page(s) on which each important word is defined and explained. That means if you want to read about, say, central lines, you can look it up in the Index and turn to the page(s) that talk about it. If you do a lot of jumping around, though, you may run into words that are unfamiliar. The Index can also be used to look up these words. The second thing is a Glossary of words that occur, but are not defined, in the text. Both the Glossary and the Index contain keys for pronouncing the words.

There are some other Special Sections at the end of the book that are for your information. The most important, and certainly the longest, is the Treatment Section. In the text, I talk about the theory of treating HIV but don't go into much detail, because the details can seem overwhelming at first. But, after a while, you'll probably have many questions about treatment—and this section will answer most of them. If you want to learn more about the body, medicine, feelings, and HIV, there is also a list of Further Readings.

One group of people may have trouble reading this book—the children. Many of you are very young and haven't had a lot of experience at reading. I hope you can find someone who is a good reader to help you (and maybe your brothers or sisters) learn about HIV. If you're younger than 10 years old, you'll need some help, but I think the person who helps you will be surprised at how well you'll understand it. After all, it's about you and that makes it pretty interesting. And there are lots of pictures to help you "see" what the words are saying.

You'll also notice that there are some blank pages in the book. These are for you to fill in, with your doctor's help. Please use these pages. I want the book to be truly yours, to grow with you, to be used in any way you wish. Whatever you want to do—color the pictures, glue in photographs, write your own thoughts, save newspaper articles—do it. That's what it's for.

Although the book is written to the child with HIV, it is also meant for others who live with, love, or work with these children. I cannot know who you are or what your relationship is to these children or whether you also have HIV. I do know that if you pretend that you are the "You" in this book, you will learn a great deal about what the child you care about is experiencing. You will also become an expert in pediatric HIV and find the words to use when talking about HIV to your child or other children—or even to adults.

You'll become an expert, because this book was written by experts. By that, I'm not talking about myself. Like you, I wasn't born knowing all this stuff, and HIV didn't exist when I went to medical school. I had to learn about it, and if I could, so can you. I thought you might like to know who my teachers were, because they are your teachers, too.

I don't have enough space here to tell you about each of them or how they helped. Maybe the best way to explain their contributions is to say that without even one of them, this book would have been less useful to you—and without some of them, it wouldn't have existed at all.

My thanks to the following organizations: The American Foundation for AIDS Research (AmFAR), The Pediatric AIDS Foundation (PAF), the Association for the Care of Children's Health (ACCH), the CDC, the U.S. Department of Health and Human Services, the National Institute of Allergy and Infectious Diseases (NAIAD), the National Cancer Institute (NCI), Project Inform, UCLA, and the Foundation for Children with AIDS.

My heartfelt thanks to these terrific people: Suzanne Rosenblatt, M.F.C.C.; Margaret Stuber, M.D.; Mark DeAntonio, M.D.; Anna Belle Kaufman; Ibby Jeppson and her colleagues at ACCH; Elizabeth Glaser; Mary Tasker, M.S.W.; Sheri Rosen, M.S., E.D.; the members of AIDS Children Teaching Us About Love (ACTUAL); E. Richard Stiehm, M.D.; Ronald Chase; September Williams, M.D.; my editor, John Dyson; the parents, faculty, and administration of the Center for Early Education; my mother, Marilyn Baker; my husband, Jean-Yves, and our children, Christopher and Cathy.

Special thanks goes to: Philip A. Pizzo, M.D., for his painstaking review of the manuscript and for boosting my spirits when I'd doubt myself; and to James Oleske, M.D., for his sensitive review, his insistence that I add a section on pain management, and his help as I wrote it. (These are the kind of doctors I would have liked to have had when I was little.)

My deepest gratitude goes to the teachers I cannot name: the families across the country who shared their insights, experiences, confusion, anger, pain, frustration, observations, discoveries—their lives—with me (and so, with you). It is through them that I learned not only what needed to be said but how to say it. If you find a sense of fun on these pages, it is because I was taught that laughter does not end where HIV begins. These families were part of this project before the writing began. They encouraged its openness and its tone. They've gone through the book page by page to keep it accurate, interesting, and real. Theirs is a truly special generosity.

All of us hope that the information in this book will be useful and that you will share it. It will always be there to answer your questions; it will never be "too busy." It won't be able to answer *all* your questions—no one book can—so we hope it also encourages you to talk to each other, to other families, to your doctors and nurses, asking questions and sharing answers about living with HIV. As one parent put it, "If I could say one thing to other parents who are HIV-positive or whose child is, let it be this: Reach out. Get involved. You're not alone in this nightmare. Get into a support network, whether it be local or national. Just get involved and speak to others like yourself. YOU DESERVE IT!"

As you reach out to each other, I hope you will also feel free to share your ideas with me. Any book, but especially one about a disease like HIV, is an ongoing process. Research is being done right now. When there is an important advance in our understanding of HIV, this book will have to be revised—so your input is important. If you have anything you'd like to share with me, please write to me at: 2001 Santa Monica Blvd., Suite 1260-W, Santa Monica, CA 90404.

I look forward to revising this book, because the future holds great promise for children and others infected with HIV. As we enter the second decade of the HIV epidemic, treatment is getting better, research is picking up, and communities are becoming more supportive and understanding of their HIV-infected members. But I'm not just talking about the faraway future, I'm also talking about the one that kids care about—the one that starts the moment after you read this. The families I worked with taught me that love, knowledge, acceptance, determination, and hope are the keys to facing *your* future with HIV—a day at a time.

LYNN S. BAKER, M.D.

You ...

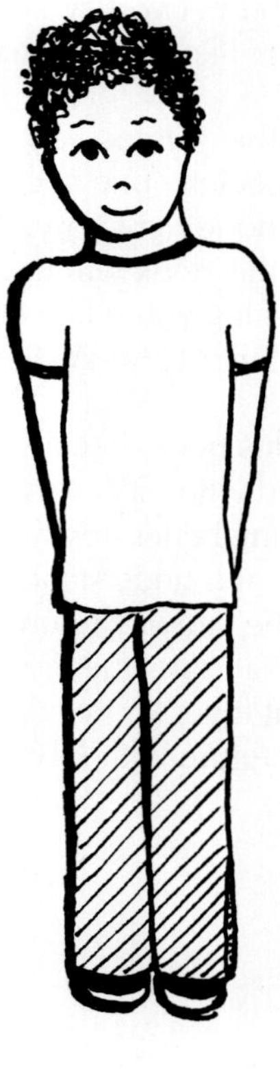

You

are very special.

That's why this book was written:

for you,

about you.

And since you are the most

important person

in this book,

this page is for your picture

and your name.

My name is____

and this is my book.

You are a person.
All people are like each other in some ways
and not alike in others.
This book was made for you by other people.
Some of them are children, like you,
who are infected by HIV, too.
They want to tell you about having HIV
so that you will know what they have learned.
Some of them are parents or caretakers
or doctors or nurses or friends, like yours.
They want to tell you what they have learned, too.
They think that if you know about HIV,
it won't be so strange to you.
And when things are not so strange
they are not so scary.

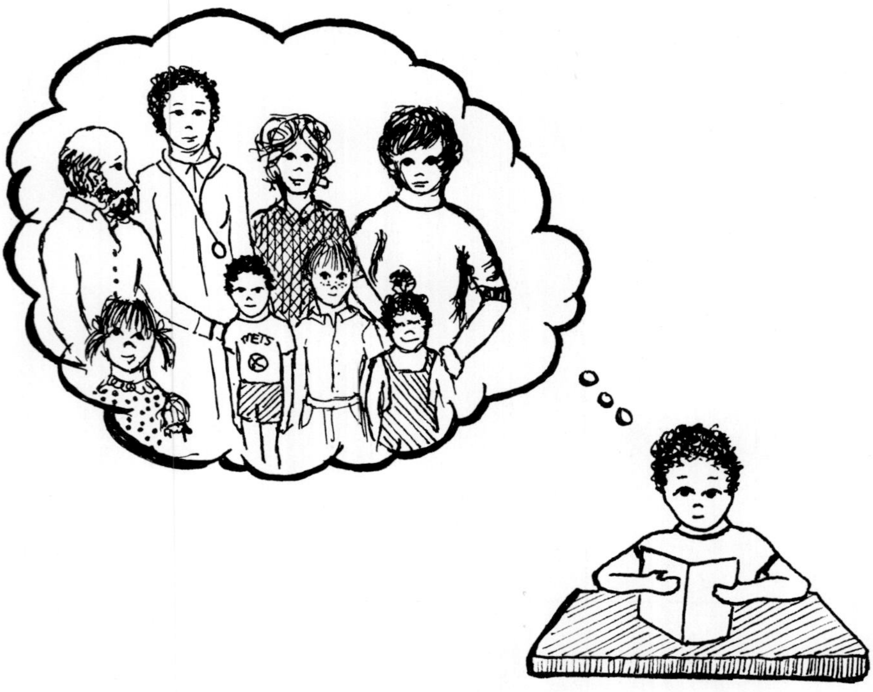

HIV can't be explained in just a few pages.
In fact, before we can even start to talk about HIV,
you have to know a lot of other things.
First, you have to know a little about your body.
Then, you need to know a lot about your immune system,
the part of your body that protects you from germs.
After you have learned about those things,
we will talk about HIV:
about what it is,
about how you got it,
about how doctors found out you had it,
about the kinds of problems it can cause,
and what will be done to try to make you better.
Later on in this book we will talk about *you* again.
About you and your life with HIV.

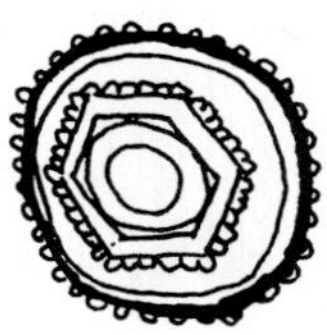

Your Body

Part of being you is being your body.
Does that sound funny?
What do you know about your body?
When you look at it, what do you see?
Skin and hair and toenails?
Arms and legs and a belly button?
When you look at your body
you only see part of it—just the outside covering.
There is an old saying that goes,
"Beauty is only skin deep."
Whoever said that must not have looked.
The part of your body that is under your skin
is as beautiful as anything can be.
Human beings are very lucky.
Not only are we bodies,
we are whole beings—
and we are able to enjoy how beautiful we all are.
Inside and out.

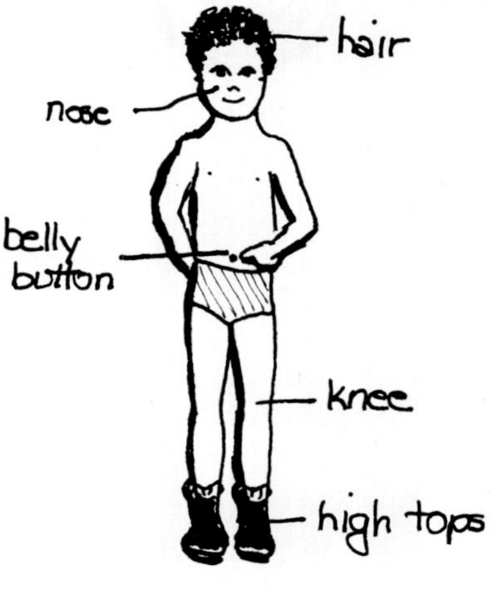

What do you think the inside of your body is like?
If you could unzip your skin and take it off,
like clothes, what would you find?
A whole new world—that's what you'd find.
It's hard to make sense of new worlds at first.
A long time ago, when doctors were learning about
what all those things are in there (anatomy),
what they do (physiology),
and what can go wrong with them (pathology)—
doctors got mixed up all the time.
But after a while they began to figure it out.
By the end of this part of the book,
you will know more about your body
than the smartest doctor did fifty years ago.

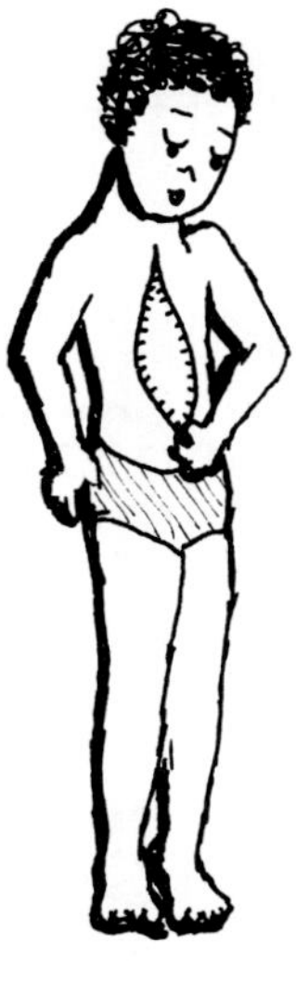

Cells

If we are going to do this right, we'd best start
at the beginning: the cell.
A cell is the smallest bit of you
that is still definitely you—
and no one else.
Here is a picture of a cell.
You probably won't think it looks much like you.
That's because you are now made
of millions of different kinds of cells.
But once upon a time, you were just one cell,
and you didn't look much like you then, either.

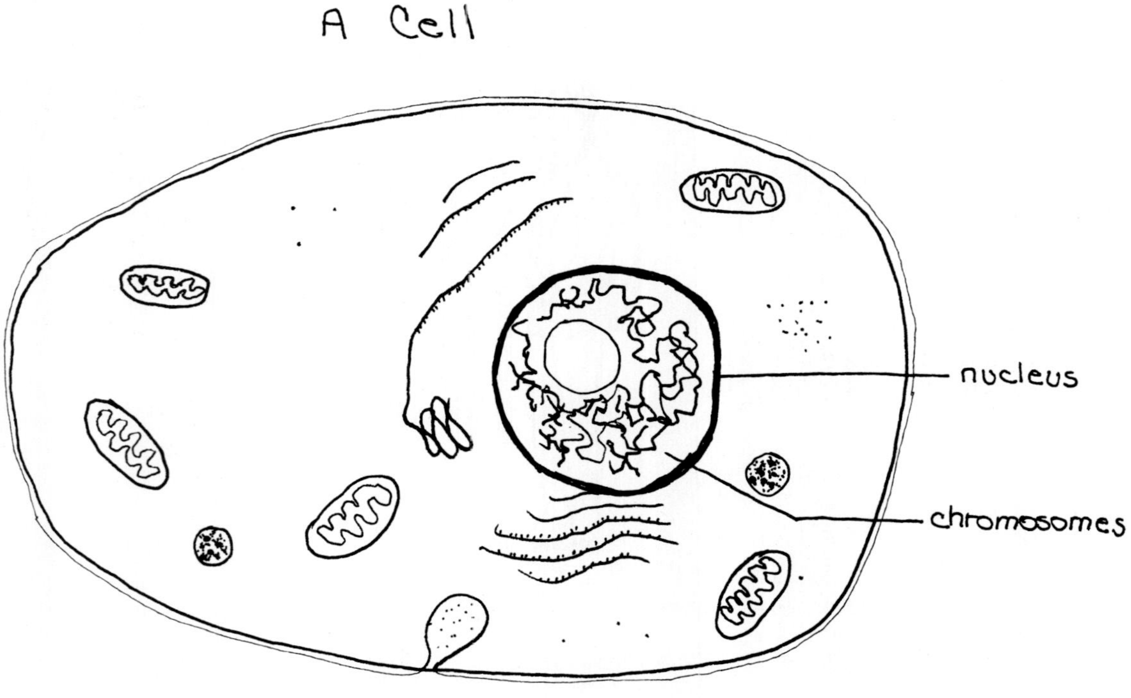

New people can only be made
when a special cell made by a man's body
(called a sperm)
combines with a special cell made by a woman's body
(called an egg, or ovum).
When your father's sperm
combined with your mother's egg,
a totally new cell was created:
the cell that would become you.

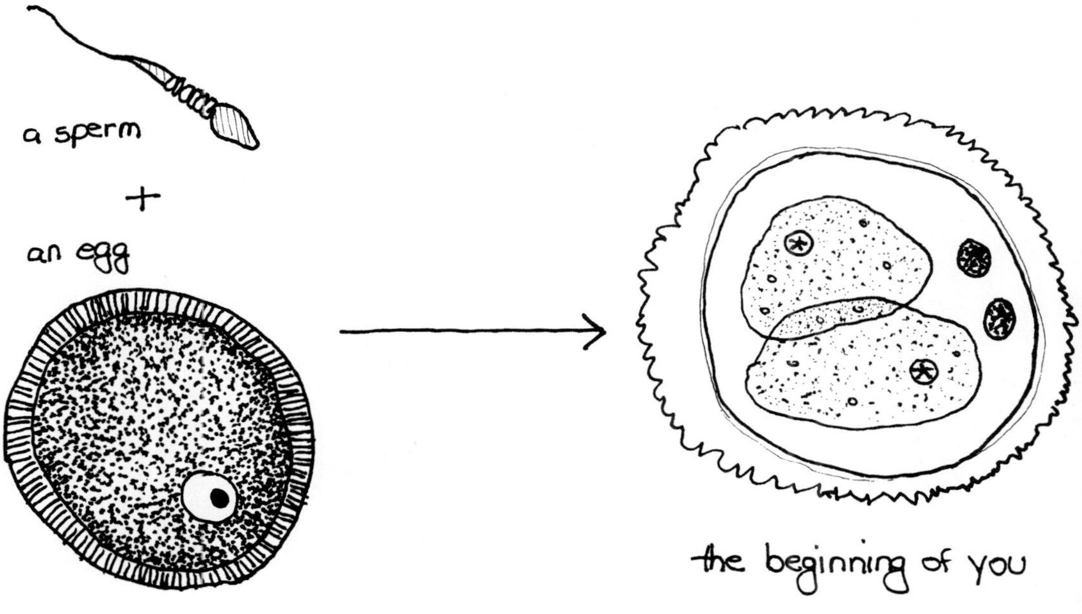

That one cell that was you
had a plan in its nucleus (its brain),
and it divided again and again
following that plan.
Some of its great-grandchildren
became liver cells,
and others became skin cells —
all according to the plan
to make you.

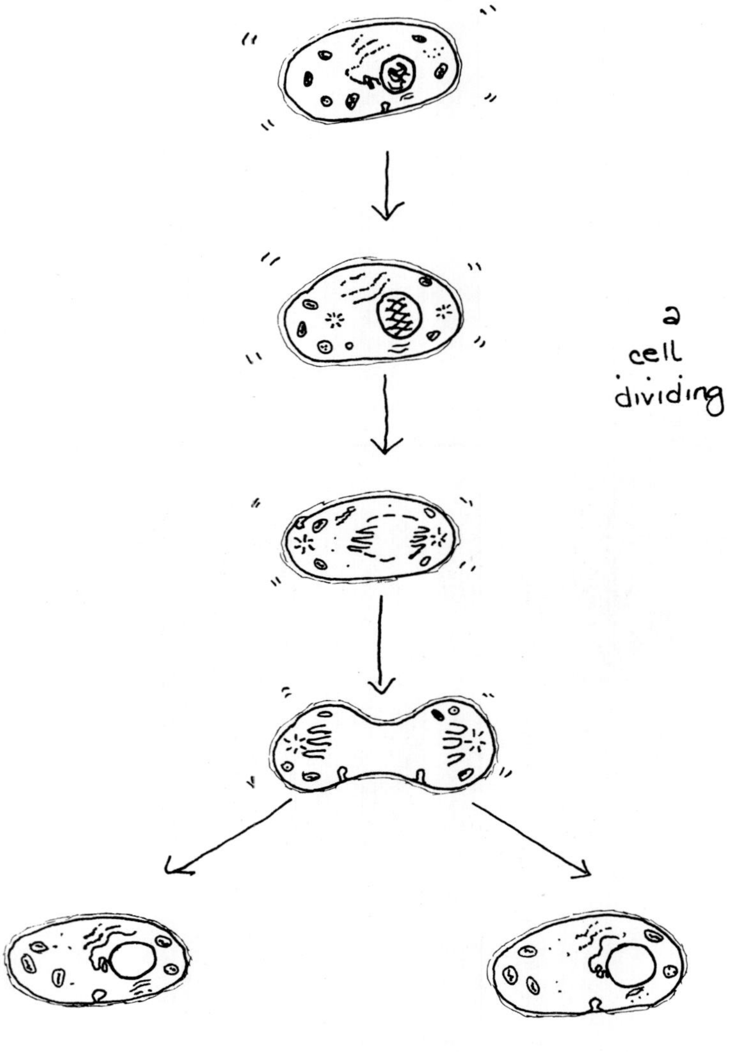

Each one of your millions of cells,
no matter how different they might seem now,
still has that same plan in its nucleus.
Each part of the plan is called a gene,
and your genes are made of long, stringy molecules
called DNA.
The plan to make you *is* your DNA.
Half of the ideas (or genes) in your DNA plan
came from your mother's egg.
The other half came from your father's sperm.
This is why you're like both of them
but not exactly like either of them.
And not at all like a giraffe or a tuna fish.
Every living being on earth
—except a few viruses—
has a DNA plan in its cells.
But you are the only living being
whose cells contain your exact DNA.

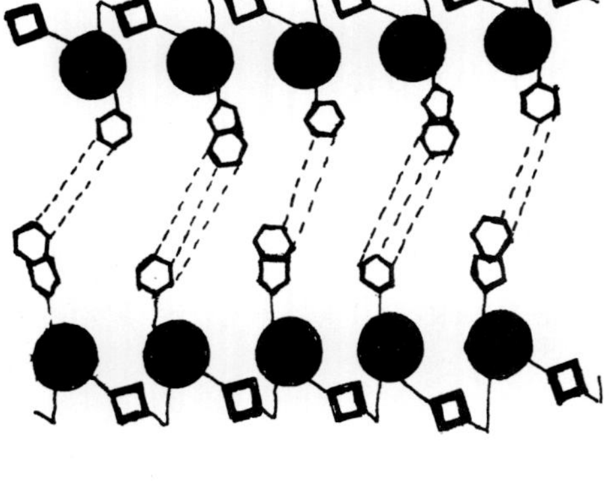

Organs and Organ Systems

Your body is made up of millions of cells,
the same way a big city is made up of millions of people.
Like people in a city, each of your cells has a job to do.
When many cells all do the same job
and they don't have to move around much to do it,
they gather in one place and work together.
The group of cells is then called an organ.
In a city, people who all do the same job organize, too—
they might all go to the same place to work,
or they might get together in labor unions.
Like people, cells often get jobs done better
when they work together.

When there is a really big job to be done,
organs get together and work with other organs.
Each organ will do a part of the work.
When organs work together like this,
they are called an organ system.
In a city, the same kind of thing happens.
Hospitals, doctors, nurses and ambulances
are all parts of the health care system.
Each group does a part of the work
for that one system.
Like groups of people, organs often get jobs done better
when they work together.

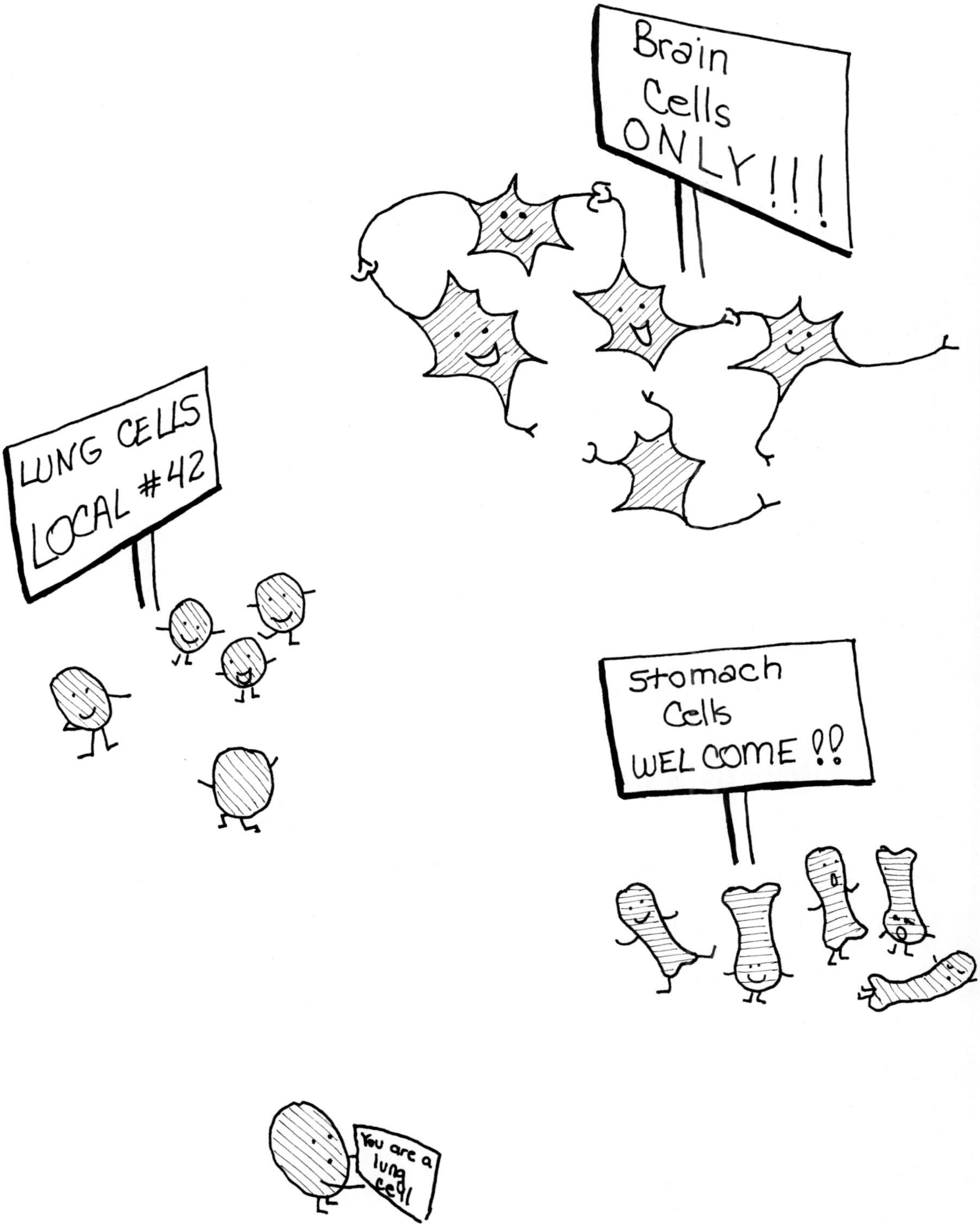
Brain Cells ONLY!!!!
LUNG CELLS LOCAL #42
Stomach Cells WELCOME !!
You are a lung cell

Your body has many organs and several organ systems.
These systems work to keep you going,
the same way that people, groups of people and systems
work to keep a city going.
What sorts of systems do you think your body—
or a city—might need?

Well, first of all, you need a supply
of food and water,
just as cities do.
That is what your digestive system is for.
Your digestive system is your body's grocery store.
Every time you eat, your digestive system works hard
to break up the food into pieces that are little enough
for your cells to use to live, work and grow.
Like people, cells need food to be healthy.

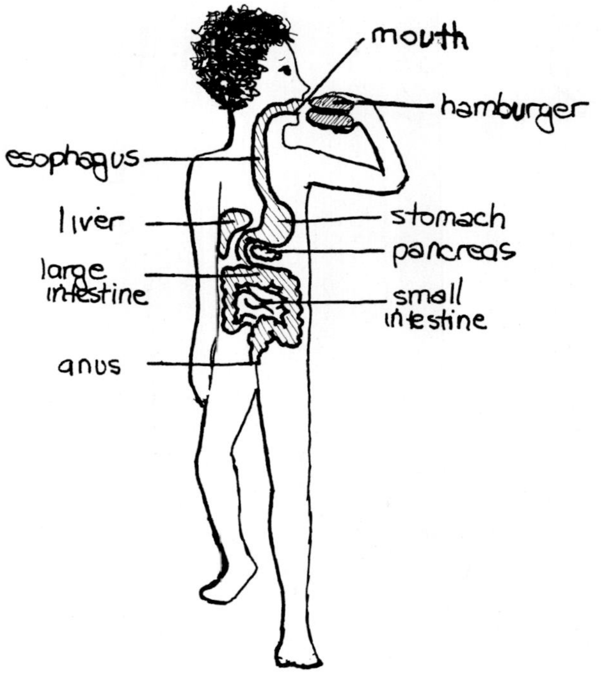

Your cells need something else from outside your body.
They need oxygen—air—and so do people in cities.
That is what your respiratory system is for.
Oxygen is a gas,
so your respiratory system is a combination
of a gas pipeline and a gas station.
Your cells need oxygen to help them burn up food
faster and better—
the same way that charcoal lighter fluid
helps you burn charcoal
faster and better.

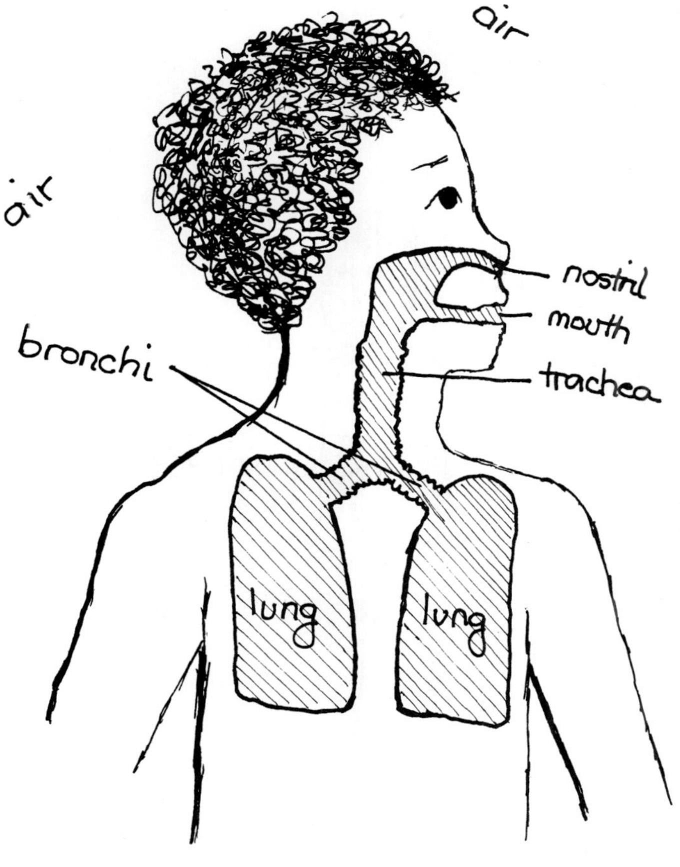

What do cells do with all the energy and materials

they get from oxygen and food?

Lots of things, like cities do.

For example, cities have factories, and so do you.

One group of your factories

is called the endocrine system.

These factories, called glands, all make hormones,

which are chemicals your entire body needs

to grow right and feel good.

Other factories are parts of other systems.

They make things that those systems need

to do their work right.

For example, some of the organs of your digestive system

make chemicals called enzymes

that break food up into little pieces.

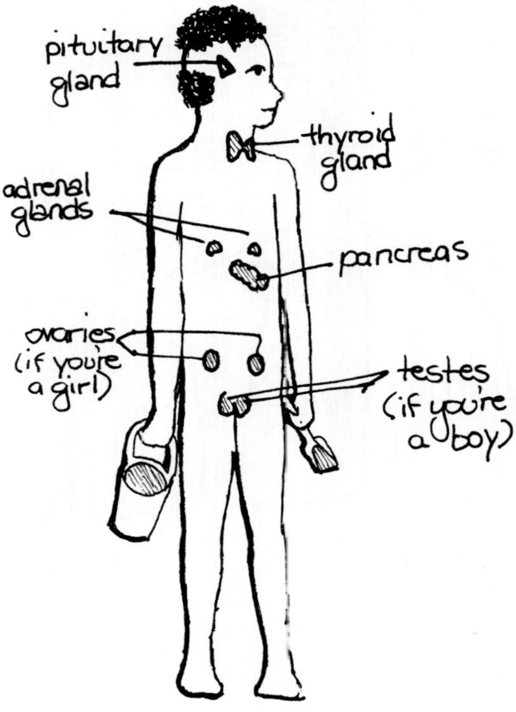

If you live in a big city,
you know that millions of people
doing zillions of things all day long
make a lot of litter and trash.
The busy cells in your body do, too.
So your body needs a system to get rid of its wastes
and recycle the good stuff.
This is what your excretory system does.
It is your body's recycling center.

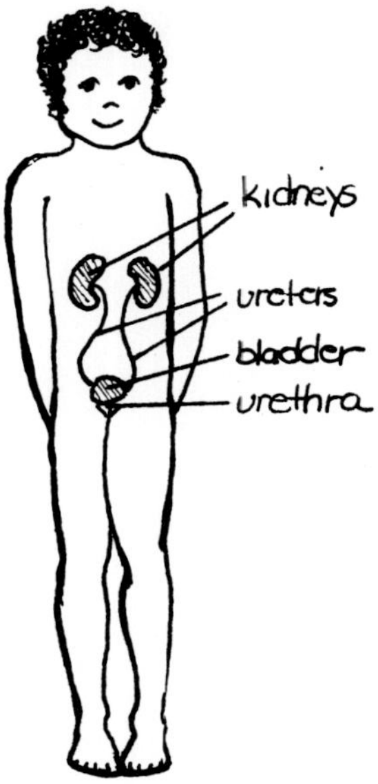

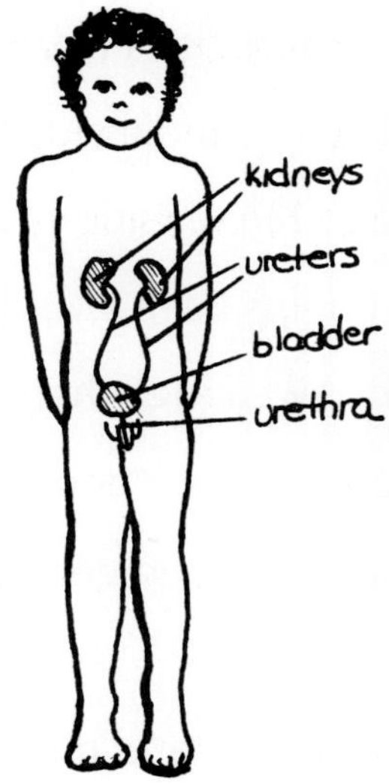

Cities have downtowns with neighborhoods around them.
Your downtown is your chest and belly,
where all of the systems we've talked about are found.
The neighborhoods are your bones and muscles.
They are another system.
Your bones protect your squishy parts and hold you up.
Your muscles help you run and walk
and breathe and talk and stick your tongue out.

Your skin is another neighborhood
and another organ system.
It is like the walls that used to be built
around cities in olden times.
It keeps the inside of you inside you
and the outside of you outside you.
It helps keep your body the right temperature
by sweating when you are too hot
and getting "goose bumps" when you are too cold.
It helps keep germs out.

Your skin and muscles and bones together
make up your city's skyline.

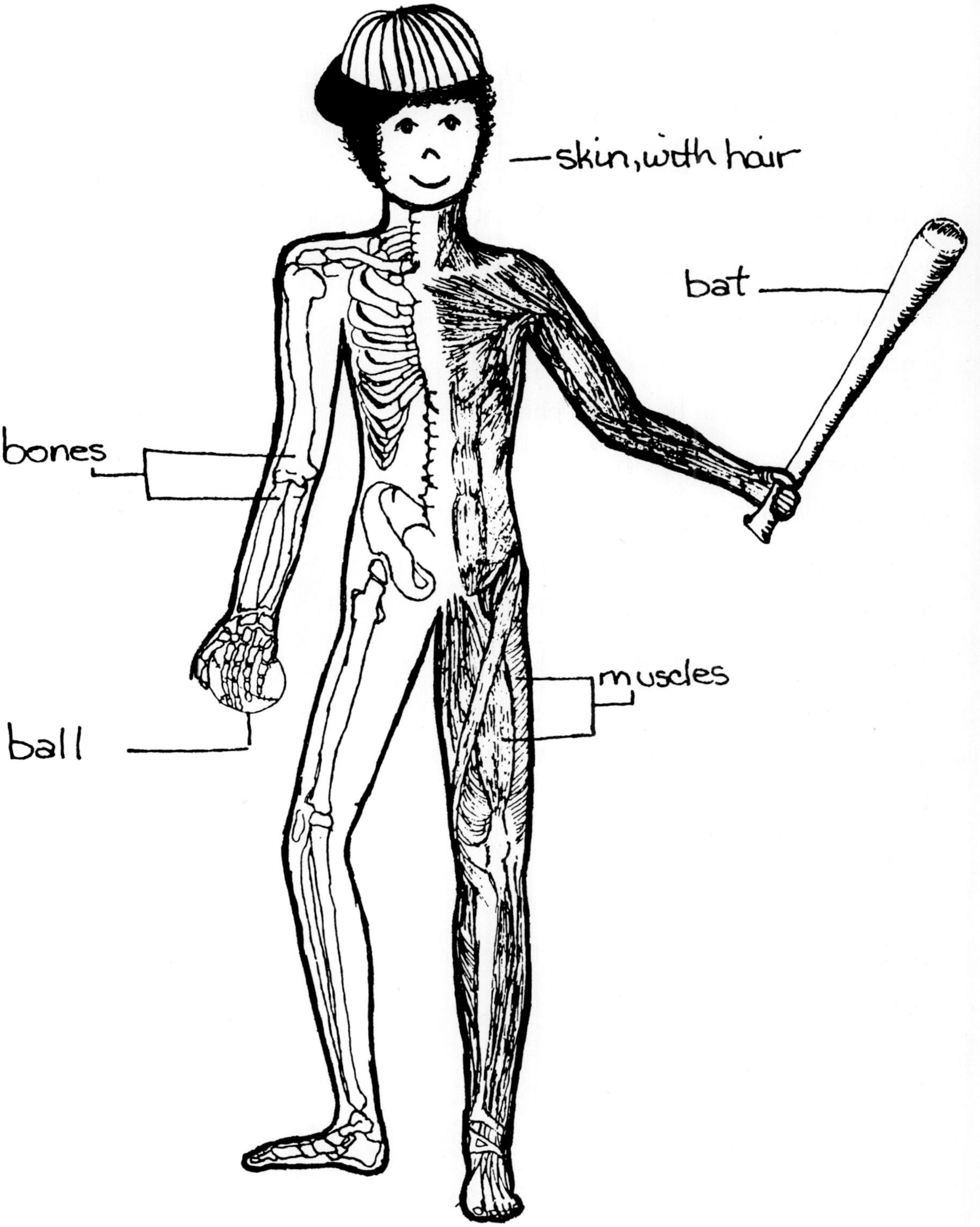
skin, with hair
bat
bones
muscles
ball

With all these cells, organs, and organ systems,
your body needs a special system
to keep all the parts working together.
This is what your nervous system does.
Your brain is kind of like your city's mayor.
It figures out what is going on and what needs to be done,
with advice from the rest of your body.
Your brain cells can "talk" with other cells
because you have telephone lines, too.
Your nerves are your body's telephone lines.
They are all over your body
the way telephone lines are all over a city.
They let the brain know what's going on in cells far away.
They let your other cells and organs know
what your brain wants them to do.
Your very own brain also does some truly special things
that only the greatest human mayors ever do.
It thinks and learns and remembers.
It hopes and dreams and imagines.
It feels feelings like happiness, sadness, or anger.
And it is your brain, not your heart, that loves.

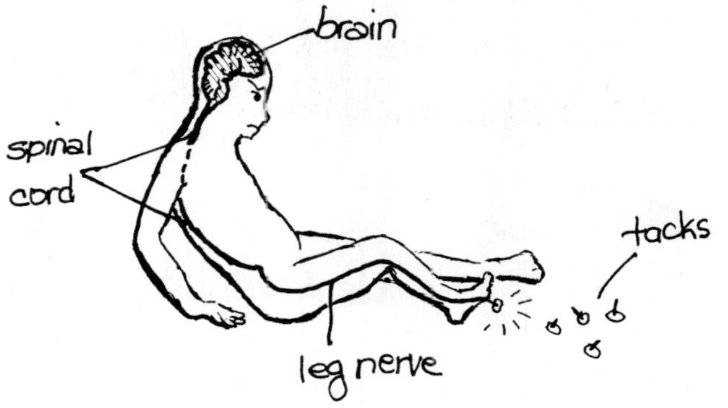

Cities need a system of roads, too.
How else can food get from your grocery store
to your table?
How else can you get things from factories?
How else can wastes get to the recycling center?
Your body's roads are called blood vessels.
They are like little, living tubes
that go to every cell in your body.
All the roads in your body are "One Way" streets:
the arteries lead away from your heart;
the veins lead back to it.
The engine that keeps everything moving on your roads
is your heart.
Together, your heart and blood vessels
are called your cardiovascular system.
If you want to feel your heart moving things
through an artery,
push gently down on the inside of one wrist
with the first two fingers of your other hand.
This is your pulse,
and it is one way you can tell
if your heart is beating steady and strong.

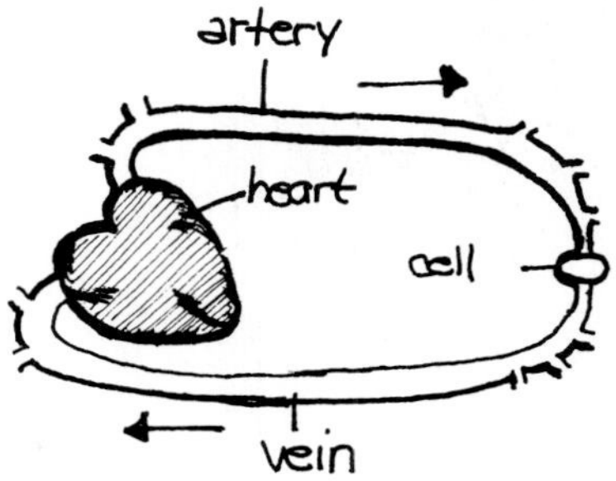

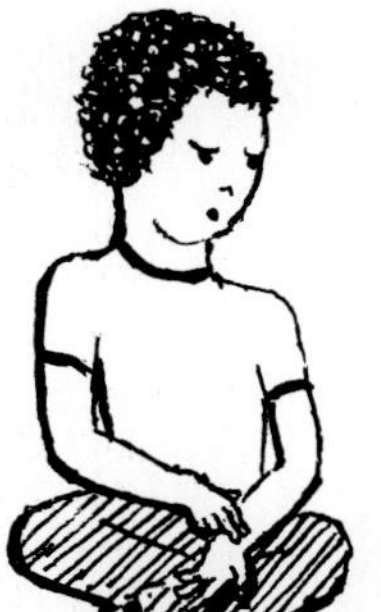

What your heart pushes along on your roads
is your blood.
Blood looks like a red liquid,
but it isn't.
It's really a pale, golden, clear liquid
with all sorts of cells and other things in it.
Some of the cells are red,
and there are so many of them that your blood looks red.
If that doesn't make sense, try this experiment.
Pour some tomato juice into a glass.
Let it sit on a shelf in the refrigerator two days.
Then look at it.
What did it look like when you put it in?
What does it look like now?
See how it is reddest at the bottom
and pale, clear and golden at the top?
That is because tomato juice
is made of tiny bits of tomato in a golden juice.
When it's all mixed up, it looks like a red liquid.
But it isn't.

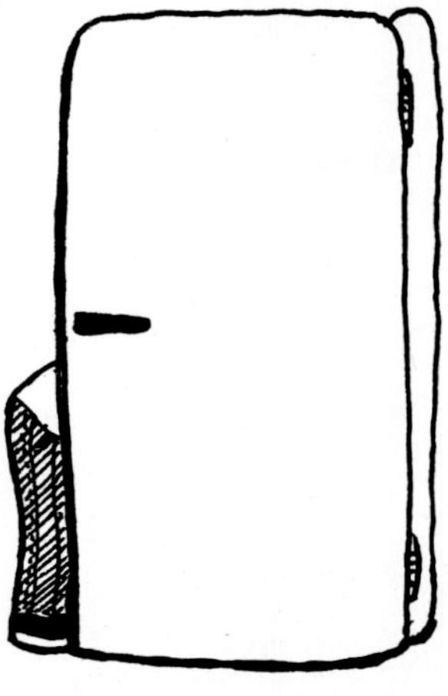

Blood is your body's transportation system.
It carries things from one cell to another
and from one part of your body to another.

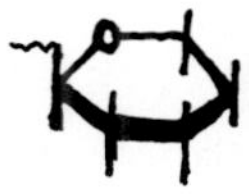

The pale, clear, golden liquid is called plasma,
and it moves all sorts of things around.
It carries teeny bits of food from your digestive system
to all your hungry cells.
It carries the things your factories make,
like hormones, to cells that use them.
It carries the wastes your cells make
to your recycling center.
And, if you get a bad infection,
it can carry germs all over your body.

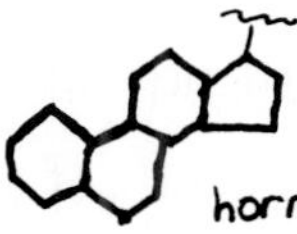

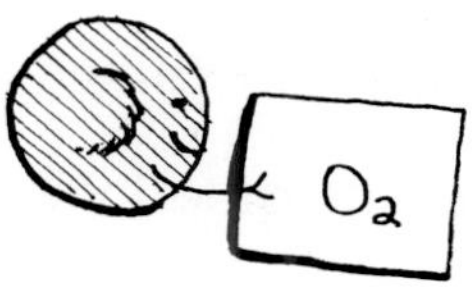

The red cells in your blood
(also called erythrocytes or RBCs)
carry oxygen from your lungs
to every cell in your body.
They get their red color
from the iron in the food that you eat.

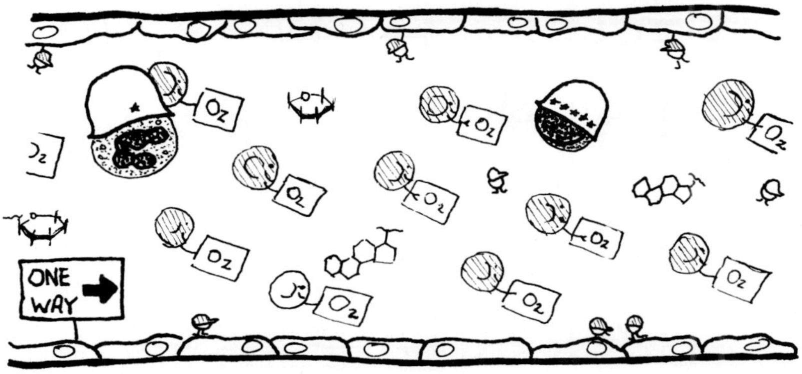

The other cells in your blood
don't carry anything around.
They have other jobs.

For example, there are many *very* teeny cells
called platelets (or thrombocytes).

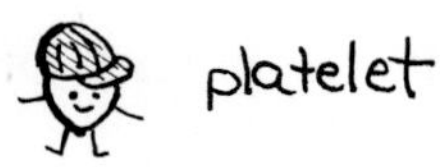

These cells may be little
but they do a big, big job.
They are your body's road repair workers.
They keep your blood vessels from leaking
and plug up the hole
(with the help of things called clotting factors)
if a vessel gets cut.

There are other cells in your blood,
called white blood cells or WBCs.

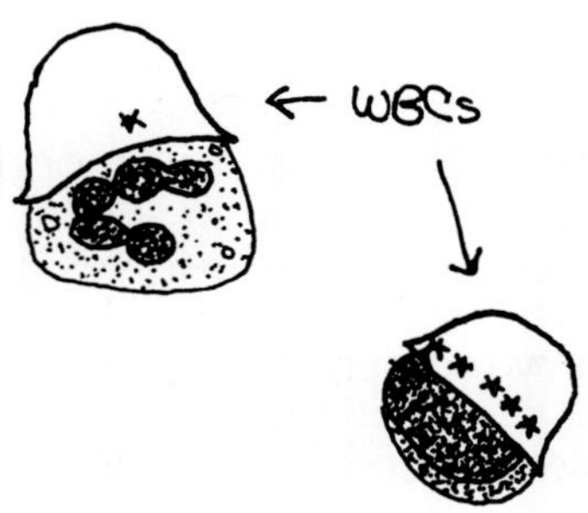

They don't carry anything around either.
They just use the blood vessel roads
to travel around your body.
You will learn what WBCs do in the next section
because they are part of your immune system.

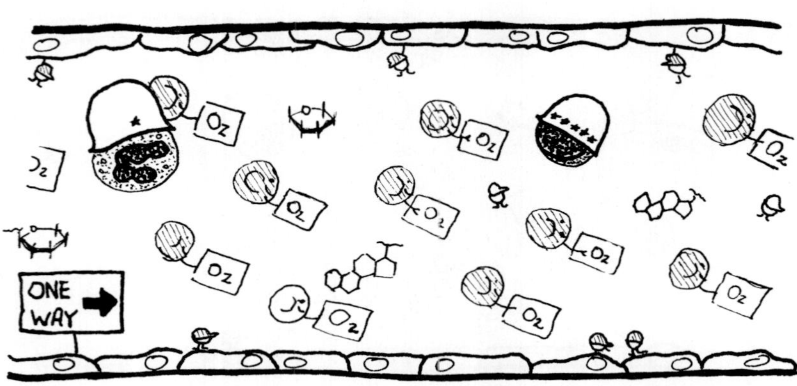

Your Immune System

We live in a world full of germs,
all kinds of germs.
Yet, most of the time
we're not even sick.
Even when we do get sick,
we almost always get better.
This is true because of our immune systems.
Cells from your immune system
are all over your body,
not just in your blood.
They are everywhere, watching for trouble.
Your immune system's job is to protect you.
It is your body's army.
It's an army that never leaves your body,
that never hurts or kills other people.
It's an army that stays home,
and it only fights when it needs to defend you.

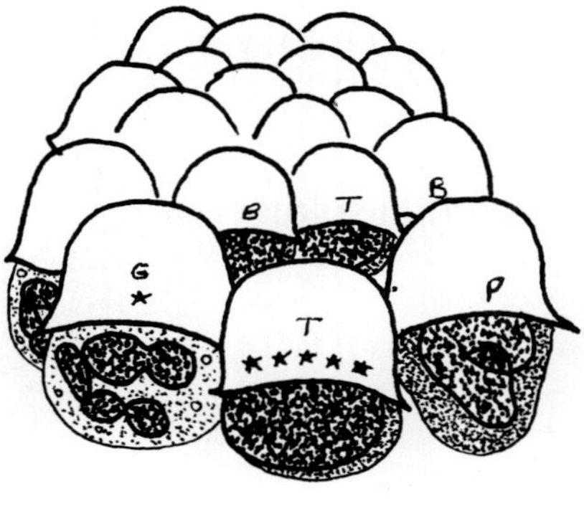

Protecting your body is a huge job.
So, like any army,
the cells of your immune system
divide up the work.
Each kind of cell
does a different kind of job.

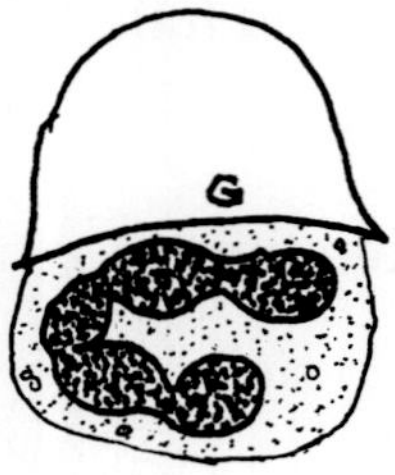

One kind of cell is called a granulocyte.
It is the best soldier you have
for fighting the group of germs called bacteria
and the diseases they cause—like strep throat.
Granulocytes defend you by surrounding bacteria
and then eating them!
Granulocytes are best at "search and destroy" jobs.

Another kind of cell is called a phagocyte.
In the blood, they are also called monocytes.
In other places, they are also called macrophages.
Phagocytes will fight any kind of germ
anywhere in your body.
They also kill germs by eating them,
but phagocytes aren't as picky as granulocytes.
They'll eat anything!
Phagocytes are your body's guerrilla soldiers.

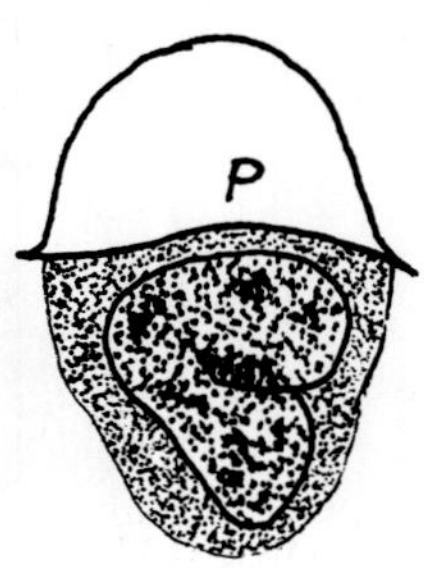

B-lymphocytes are another kind of cell.
Most of the time, B-lymphocytes, or B-cells,
don't do much but hang around in lymph nodes
(which are sort of like army bases).
But when a germ gets inside your body
and your B-lymphocytes hear about it,
they do something really amazing:
they change into completely different cells
called plasma cells.
Plasma cells are like factories.
They make sticky things called antibodies
that float around in the blood
and stick to any germs they get near.
Antibodies are like signs that tell other WBCs,
"This is an enemy. Get it!"
Those antibody signs really help
the other immune cells do their jobs.
B-lymphoctyes, and therefore plasma cells,
are best at being scouts.

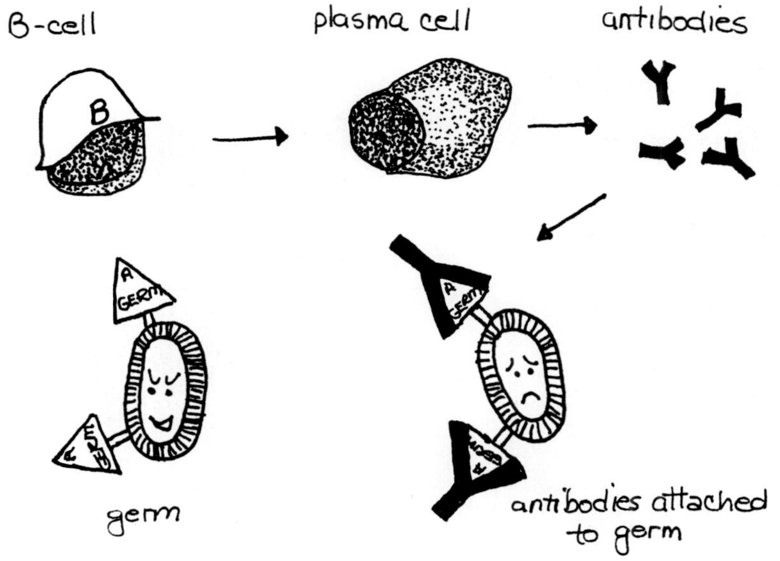

T-lymphoctyes, or T-cells,
are the most important kind of cell
in your immune system.
They are not only soldiers
(they do best at fighting germs
like viruses and funguses)—
they are also commanders.
They're the ones that tell B-lymphocytes
to turn into plasma cells.
They send chemical orders to other cells,
telling them where the trouble is
and what to do when they get there.
Some T-cells join special commando teams
that kill cells that have germs
hiding inside them.
Other T-cells are called "helper T-cells"
because their main job is helping
all the other immune cells get their jobs done.
Still other T-cells have the job of remembering
every germ that's ever been inside your body.
T-cells are the smartest cells
in your immune system.
Maybe in your whole body.

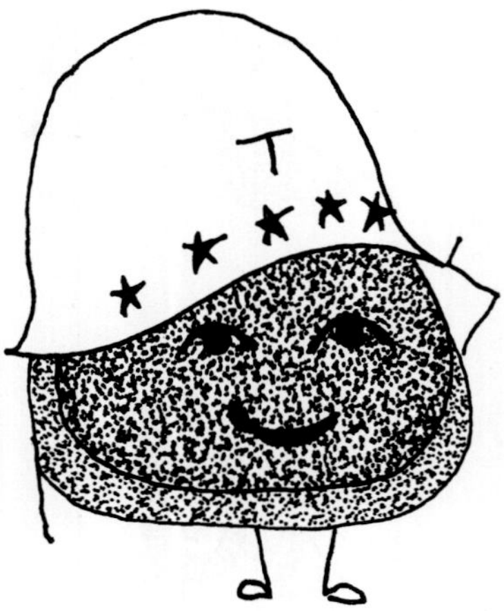

Like you, your T-cells were born smart.
But also like you,
your T-cells didn't start out knowing very much.
They needed to learn a lot
if they were going to protect you.
The first thing they needed to learn
was how to tell the difference
between cells that are part of your body
and cells (and other things) that aren't.
How do they do this?
After all, everyone's cells
look pretty much the same to us.
They can do it because everyone's cells
don't look at all the same to T-cells.
It turns out that each of your cells
has special markers on it,
sort of like labels.
These labels are called antigens.
Every cell in your body
has an antigen label on it,
and many cells have more than one.

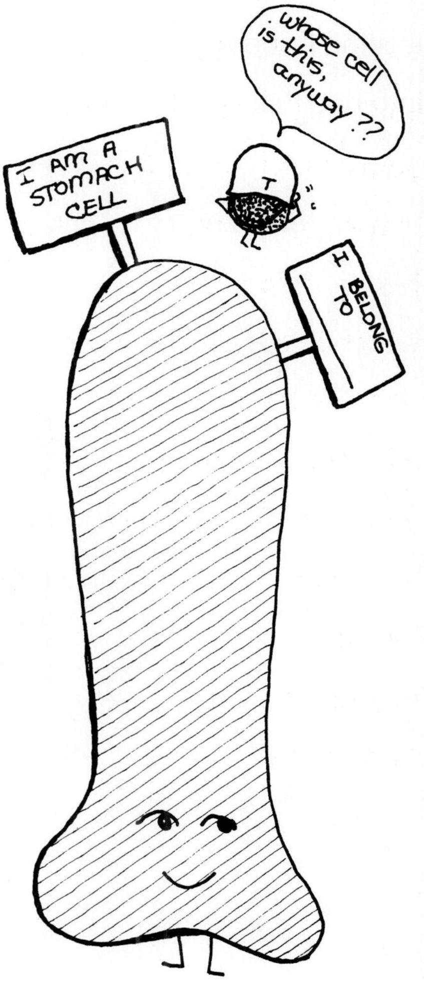

Helper T-cells, for example,
have at least three antigen labels.
One of them says, "I am a T-cell."
Another says, "I am a helper"
(the official name for this one is the CD-4 antigen).
The third says, "I belong to ________________________ "
(you can write your name in the blanks,
if you want to).
The first two antigens are found
on everybody's helper T-cells.
It is the last one that turns any old helper T-cell
into one that is yours alone.

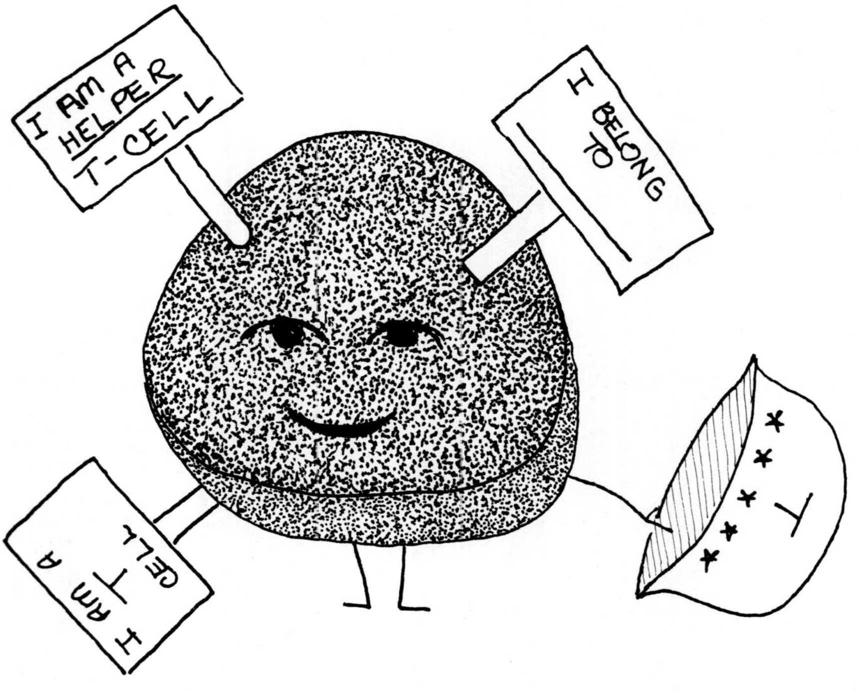

By the time you were born,
your T-cells had memorized
every antigen on every single one of your cells.
Your T-cells know what's *you* and what's not
better than any person does.
Even your best friend.
By the time you were born,
your T-cells have also been to school
in a place called your thymus gland.
There they learned everything they needed to know
to be the commanders for your immune system.
When a cell from your immune system
sees another cell with your antigens on it,
it will leave that cell alone.
But when it sees a cell
with someone else's antigens on it
(or some*thing* else's antigens on it,
like a germ's),
your immune system will do everything it can
to destroy the strange cell
and protect you from harm.

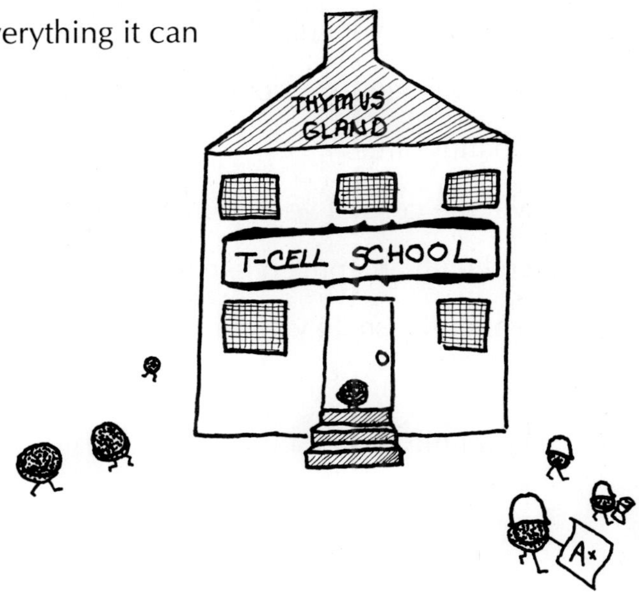

When all the parts of your immune system
are working right and working together,
you are pretty much protected against germs.
You never even know
about most of the germs that get inside you
because they're not around long enough
to make you feel sick.
Even sneaky germs,
the ones that try to hide from your immune system
by going *inside* your cells
instead of just going around and between them,
are almost always found and destroyed.
Sneaky germs get found out
because they make the cell they live in sick
and sick cells don't look like healthy cells.
Sick cells have different antigen labels on them,
antigens made by the germ inside them.
Instead of saying something like,
"I am one of your liver cells,"
the sick cell's antigens say something else, such as,
"I am a hepatitis virus."
No way will the cells of your immune system
ignore a cell with an antigen like that!
They'll go after the sneaky germs,
and they'll get them.
It just takes a little longer.

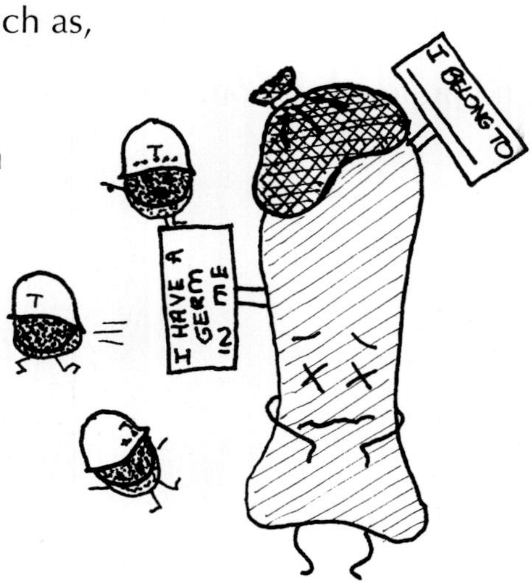

Your immune system is truly amazing.
It knows you better than anyone
and protects you better than anything,
as long as it is working properly.
The things you and your parents and your doctor do
to protect you from germs—
like eating healthy foods,
staying clean,
getting enough sleep
and taking medicines—
only help your immune system do its job better.
Its job of protecting you.

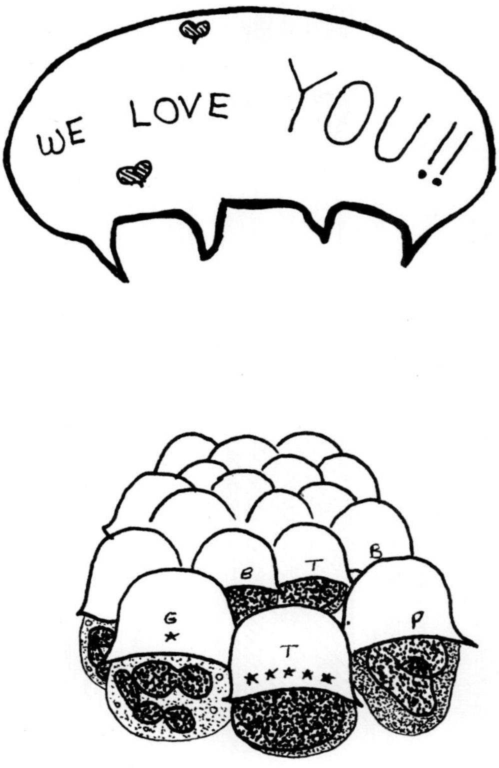

At the beginning of this part of the book,
we said that you are very special.
That in all this world
there is only one you.
Now that you know more about your body,
about your DNA
and especially about your immune system,
you know we weren't just saying that
to make you feel good.
We said it because it's true.

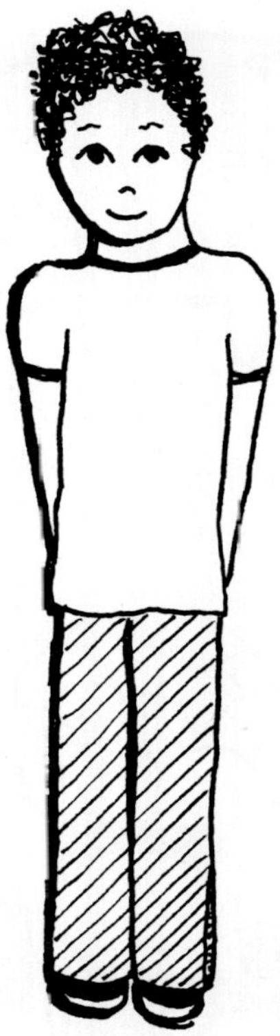

... And HIV

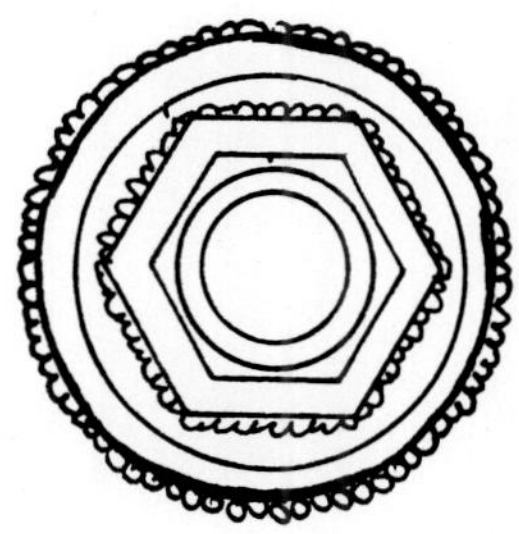

What Is HIV?

It's easy to answer this question.

What's hard is understanding the answer.

HIV stands for

"**H**uman

Immunodeficiency

Virus,"

but it takes so long to say that

that most people just say, "HIV," instead.

"Human" means people.

"Immunodeficiency" means

an immune system that doesn't work right.

A "virus" is a kind of germ.

So, when people talk about HIV,

they are talking about the virus

that makes people's immune systems sick.

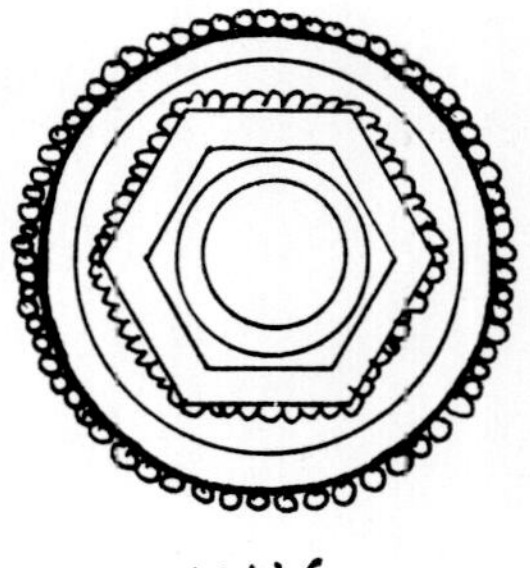

HIV

What Are Viruses?

In order to understand
what HIV is,
you need to know something
about viruses and other germs.
Germs are little, teeny living things.
They are so small you can't even see them
unless you have a microscope,
and even then you still can't see some of them.
There are zillions of kinds of germs,
and they live all over the world.
Most germs don't bother people much.
The germs that do make people sick
probably don't really mean to.
They just happen to enjoy living in our bodies,
or they end up living there by accident.
We don't get sick every time
a germ gets into our bodies,
because of our immune systems.
Only when lots and lots of germs get into us,
or when our immune system isn't working right,
are most germs able to make us sick.

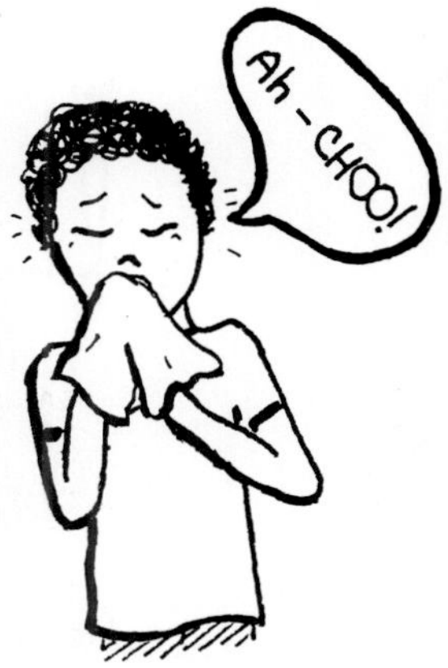

When you look at a germ through a microscope
(ask your doctor to show you some),
you'll see that most of them
look a lot like cells
only smaller.
That's because most of them *are* cells,
only they are very small cells.
And instead of each cell being
one part of a bigger being
(as each of your cells is one part
of your whole self),
one germ cell
is one whole germ.

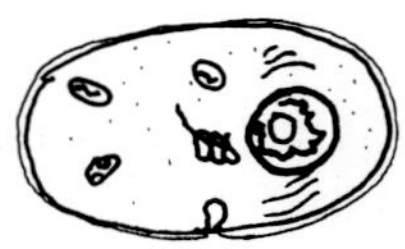

a human cell

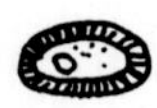

a bacteria cell

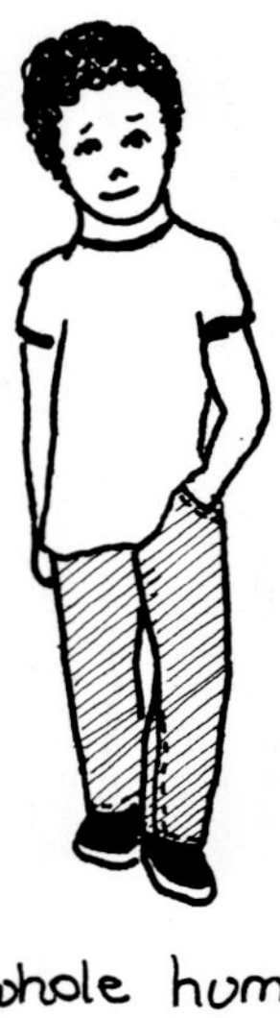

a whole human being

a whole bacteria

The kinds of germs that are like tiny cells are:

bacteria (they cause diseases like strep throat),

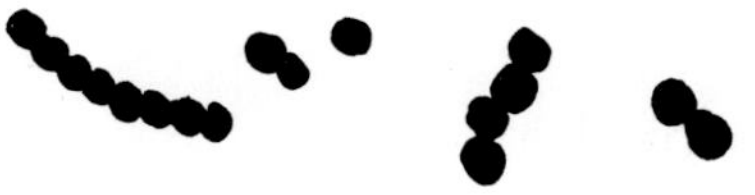
Each little ball is one
Strep germ, but they
like to get together
making pairs and chains

fungi (they cause diseases like thrush),

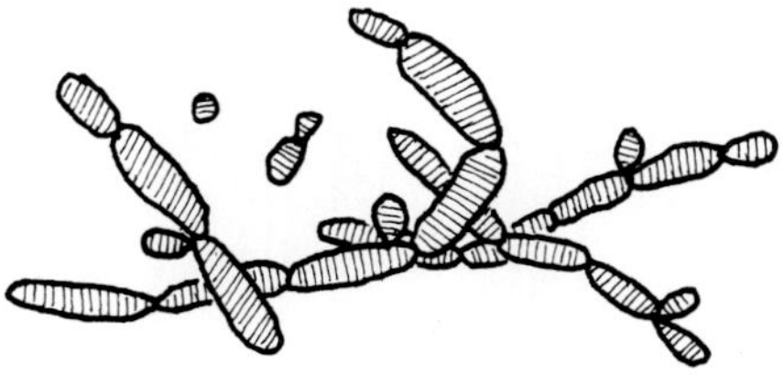

and some parasites (they cause diseases like toxoplasmosis).

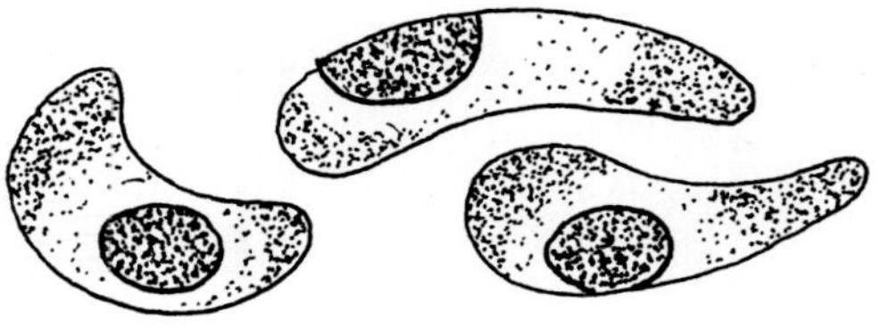

These cell-like germs
are a lot like our own cells.
They need food.
They grow—which they do by dividing—
just as our cells do.
They can get sick,
and they can die.
Life is kind of the same
whether you're one of these cell-like germs
or a regular cell—
or even a person.

Life is very different for viruses.
Viruses don't look like cells,
and they don't act like cells.
They don't look like cells
because viruses are much, much smaller,
and they don't have room inside them
for all the things that cells have.
Here is a picture of some viruses.
What do you think they look like?
Machines? Spaceships? Crystals?
Aliens? Mummies? Igloos?

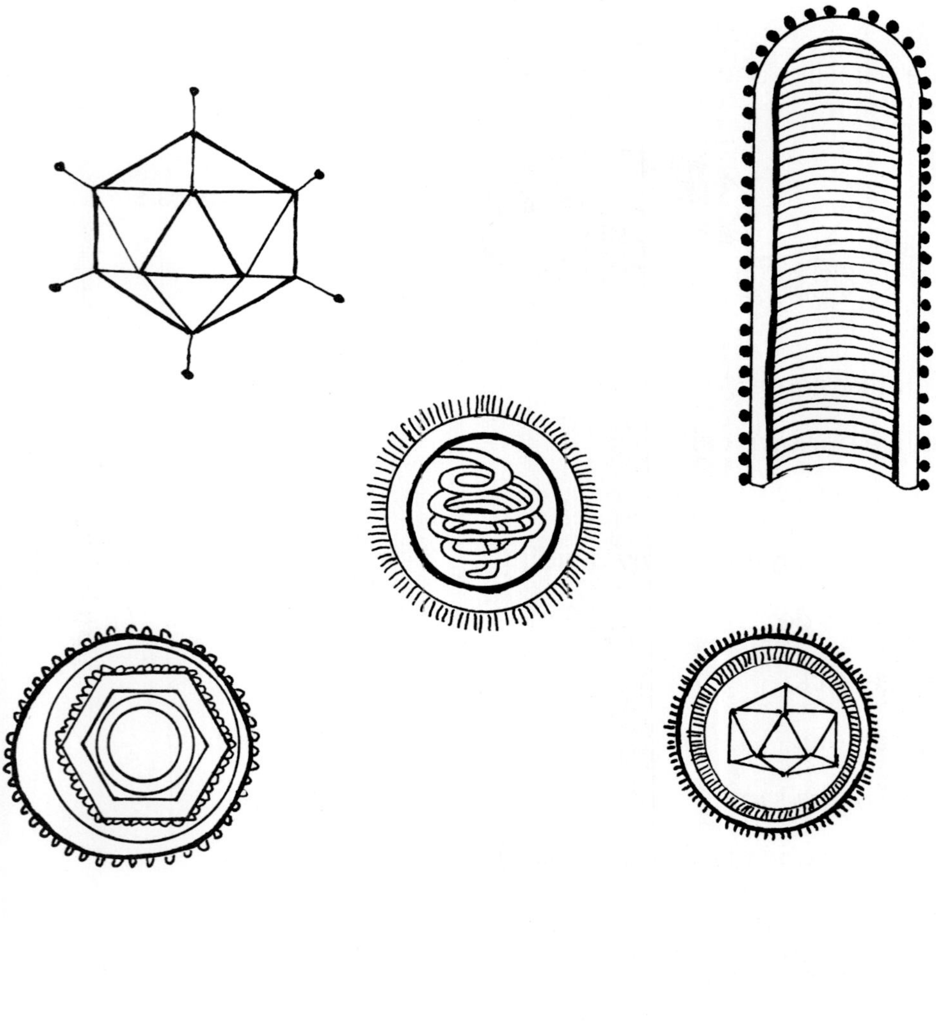

Their smallness is also the reason
that viruses don't act like cells.
They just can't.
They don't have enough parts.
They don't eat.
They don't grow.
They don't get sick.
They don't even die
(although they can be "inactivated,"
which is kind of like being dead).
The only thing a virus has
that other germs and cells also have
is a string of DNA
(or something like it called RNA),
which is a plan to make new viruses.
And the only thing a virus does
that is anything like what other living things do
is reproduce, which means make new viruses.

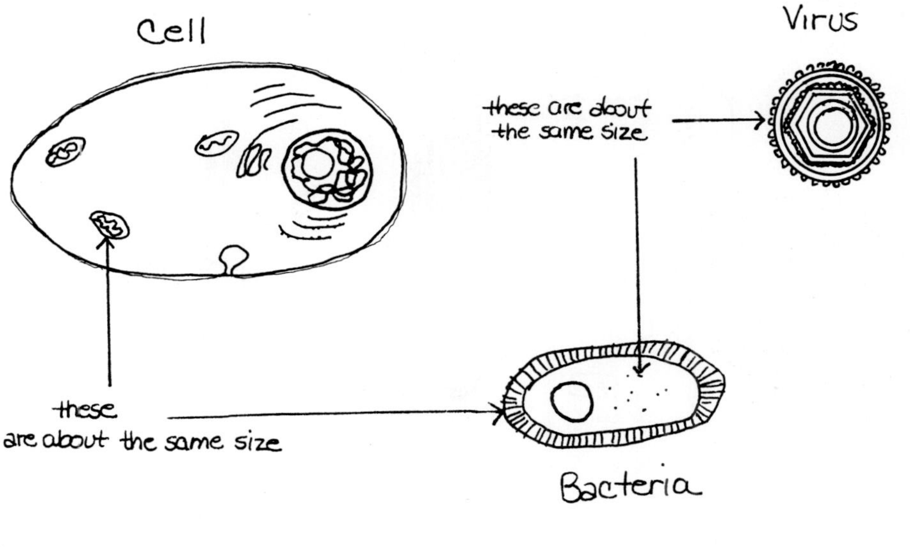

People reproduce by having babies.
Cells and cell-like germs reproduce by dividing.
Viruses are too small to have babies
and even too small to divide.
A virus is really just
a tiny DNA or RNA plan to make more viruses
all wrapped up in a protein coat.
A virus is sort of like a video game,
full of information and ideas
but unable to do anything at all
until it's put into a video game machine.
The thing a virus needs to get into, though,
is not a machine, but a living cell.
Only in a living cell will it get the energy,
the equipment, and the materials it needs
to make new viruses.

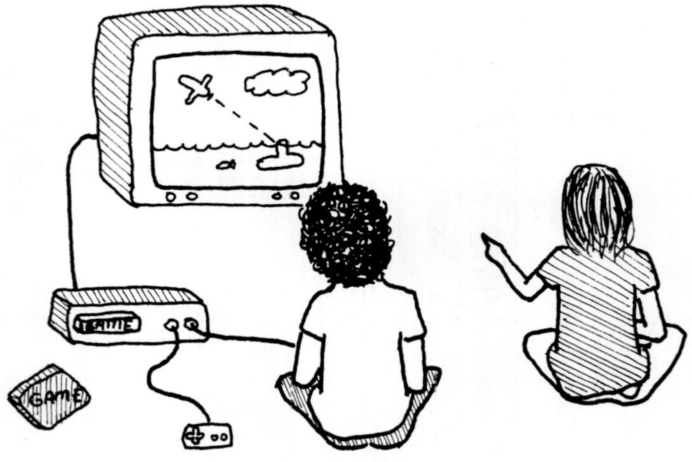

What happens when a virus infects a living cell
is sort of like what would happen
if the president of a factory
that builds airplanes
suddenly got infected
by the idea of making toy cars.
The president would have all the parts needed
to build toy cars.
By changing a few things in the factory,
toy cars could actually be made.
The problem is
that the factory is supposed to make airplanes—
not toy cars.

A cell infected by a virus
stops doing what it's supposed to do
and turns into a virus factory.

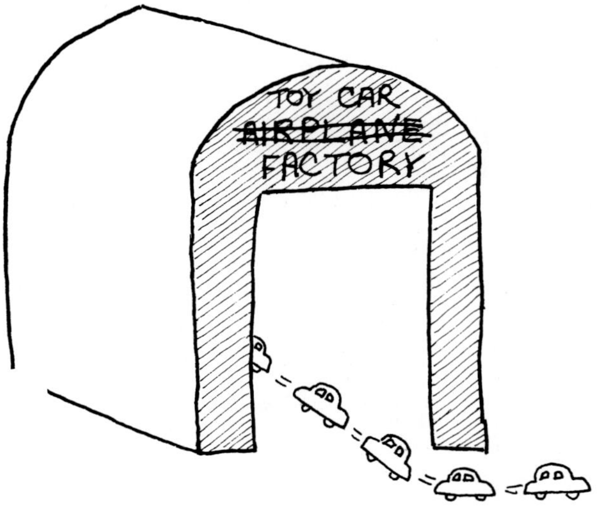

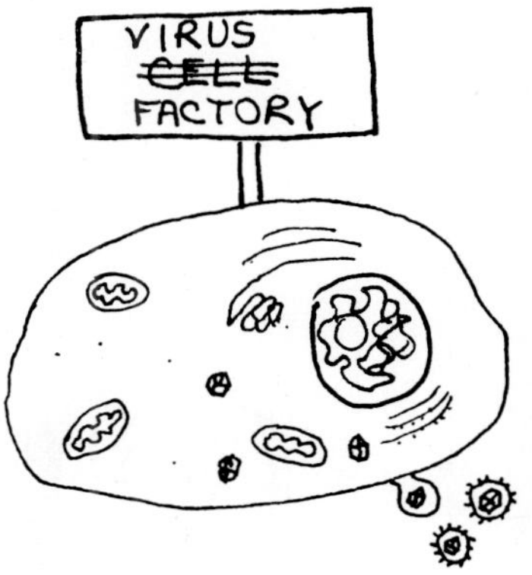

All viruses cannot infect all kinds of cells.
Each virus is specially designed
to infect only certain kinds of cells.
Viruses can tell one kind of cell from another
the same way T-cells do:
using the cell's antigens.
Viruses can tell one cell's antigens from another's
by using its own antigens.
If you think of a *virus's* antigen as being a *key,*
and a *cell's* antigen as being a *keyhole,*
you can imagine how this works.
The virus goes around sticking its antigen key
into every cell antigen keyhole it can
until it finds one that fits.
Then, the virus's key turns in the cell's keyhole
opening a tiny door into the cell,
and the virus goes right in.

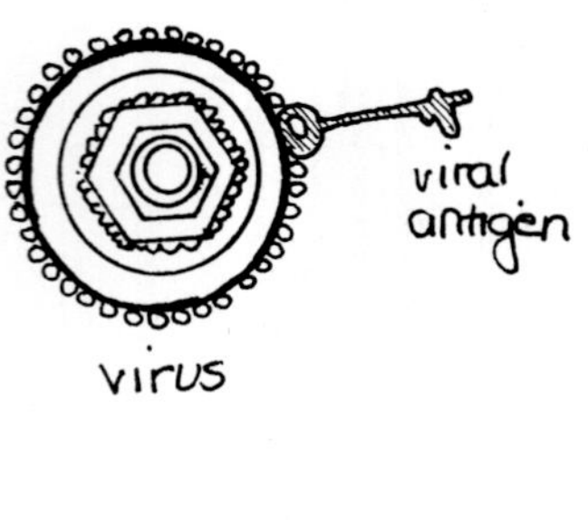

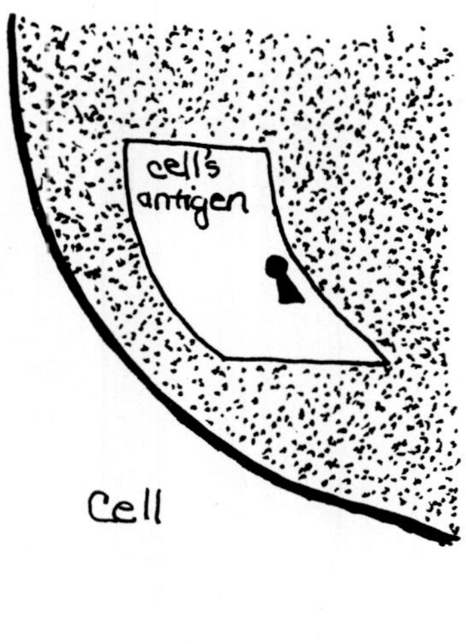

Once inside,
the virus gets rid of
whatever is left of its protein coat.
Then it's not even a virus anymore.
It's just a piece of DNA or RNA.
Cells can't tell the difference
between their own plans
—their own DNA or RNA—
and someone else's ideas,
like a virus's DNA or RNA.
That's why the cell starts making viruses.
It makes viral DNA or RNA.
It makes viral proteins.
It makes viruses
until all the stuff in the cell is used up.
Then, the cell kind of explodes
throwing out thousands of viruses
and killing itself.
To make matters even worse,
some viruses even steal bits of the cell's covering
to make their own outer coats fancier.
Some thanks the cell gets.

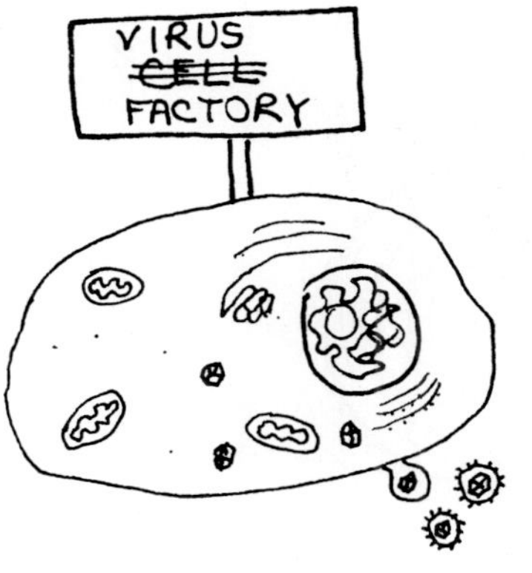

Viruses are all work and no play,
so they live very dull lives.
But viruses are also nearly perfect germs.
They hide inside living cells,
including our own,
and turn them into virus factories.
Like creatures from the Land of Oz,
they can never die,
but they *can* be destroyed.
Heat and certain chemicals can destroy many viruses.
So can our immune systems,
if they're working properly.

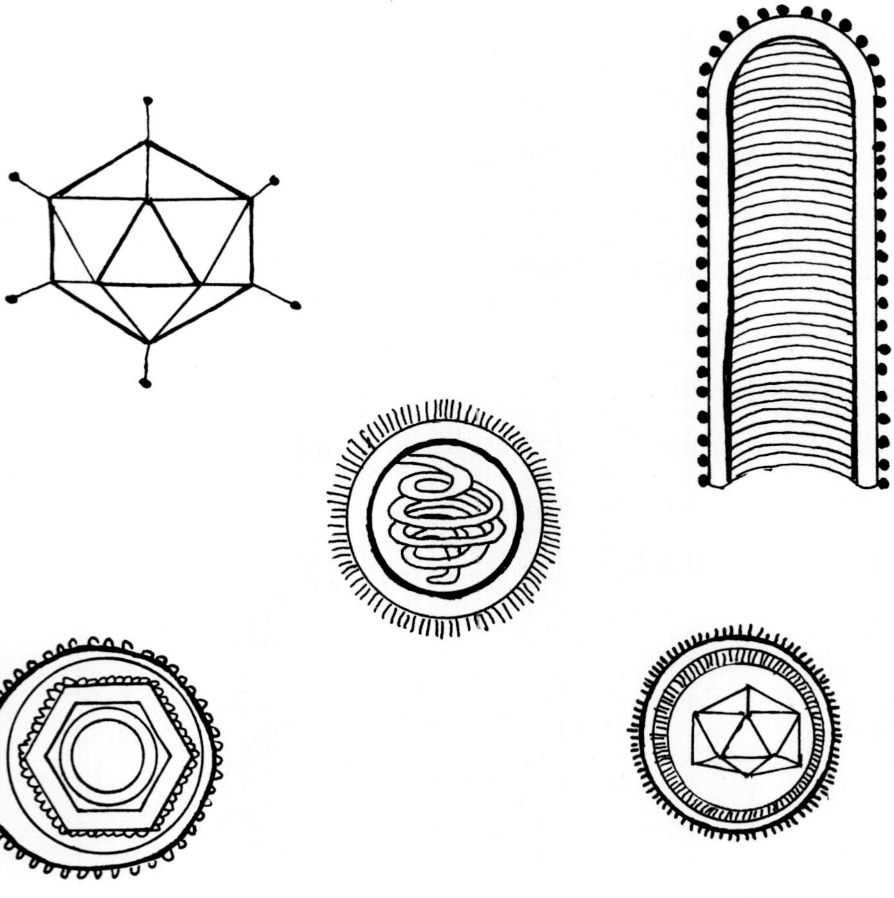

What Is Immunodeficiency?

Not everyone's immune system
works properly.
When a person's immune system
is not working properly
that person has an immunodeficiency.

The kinds of problems a person
with an immunodeficiency will have
depend on what part of the immune system
is deficient.
"Deficient" can mean either
that a part of the immune system is missing,
or that it is there but not working very well.

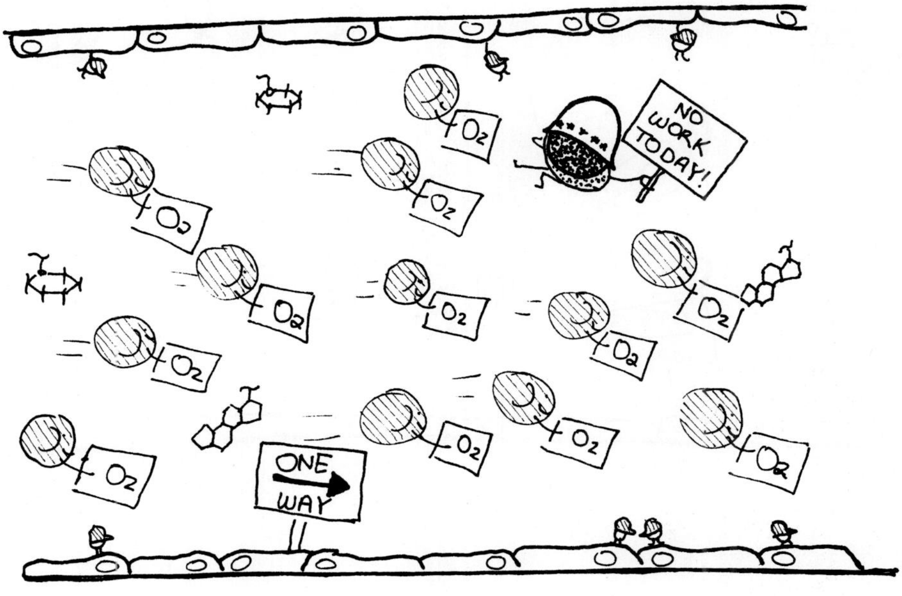

There are many different kinds
of immunodeficiency,
depending on which part of the immune system
is sick or deficient.
Sometimes just one part of the immune system is sick.
Sometimes many parts are sick at the same time.
HIV is an example of something
that can make many parts of the immune system deficient.
But, no matter what causes an immunodeficiency,
the results are the same.
The person gets more infections,
and these infections are more serious
and last longer than they otherwise would.

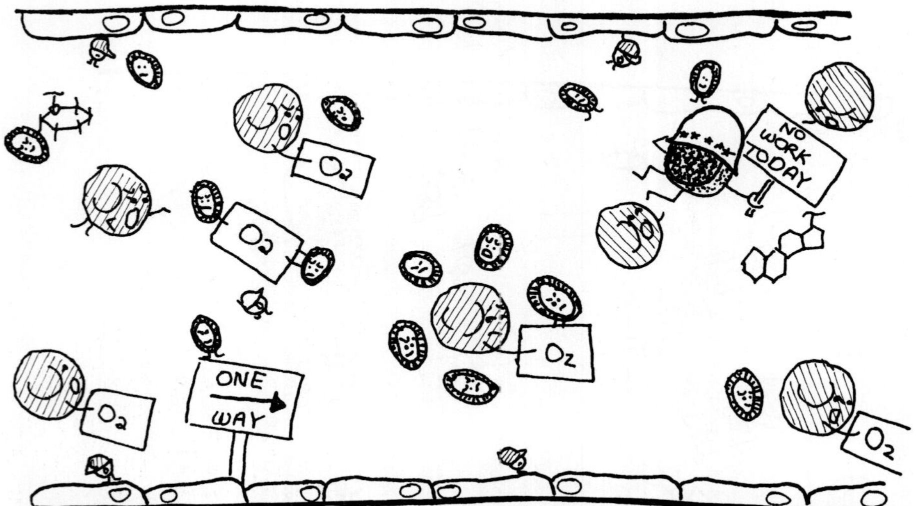

How Does HIV Cause Immunodeficiency?

Now that you know what HIV *is,*
you need to learn what it *does*
and how it does it.

In most ways,
HIV is like many other viruses.
It has a fancy protein coat
and an RNA plan for new viruses.
Like all viruses,
it needs to find a living cell
that it can get inside
and turn into a virus factory.
What makes HIV different
from *most* other viruses
is that it likes best to infect helper T-cells.
What makes HIV different
from *all* other viruses
is that it kills helper T-cells.

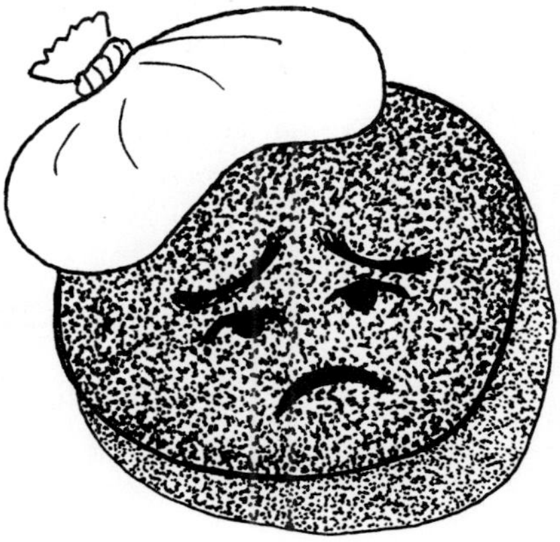

When HIV first gets inside a person's body,
it does what any other virus would do:
it tries to find a cell
with an antigen keyhole
that its own antigen key will fit.
The antigen keyhole it is looking for
is the CD-4 antigen,
which is the antigen that makes a helper T-cell
look different from other T-cells.
If the HIV finds a helper T-cell
(which isn't hard because they're found
everywhere in the body),
the HIV will put its antigen key
into the CD-4 keyhole,
open a tiny door in the cell's "skin,"
and go right in.

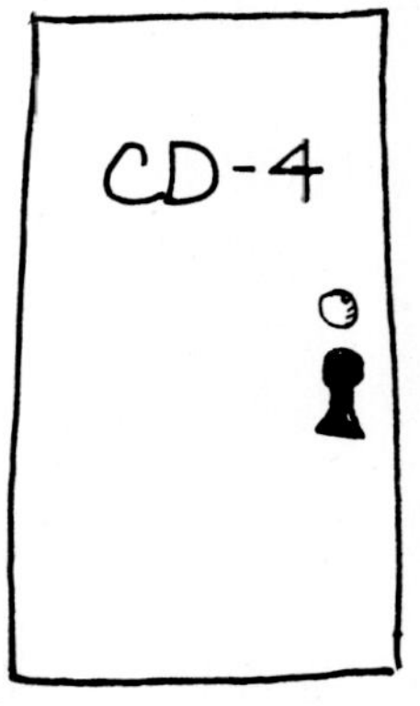

Once inside,
it gets rid of whatever's left of its protein coat.
One of the pieces of that coat
is an enzyme called reverse transcriptase.
An enzyme is something that is needed
to either break chemical things up
or put chemical things together.
Reverse transcriptase is the put-together kind.
It puts together some DNA using the viral RNA as a model.
The DNA it puts together is called "proviral DNA,"
because it will later be used to make new viruses.
This proviral DNA goes into the helper T-cell's nucleus
and mixes itself up with the cell's own DNA.
The plan to make more HIV
becomes a part of the cell's own plan.
Sometimes, the proviral DNA gets right to work
and turns the helper T-cell into a virus factory,
making new viruses and killing the helper T-cell.

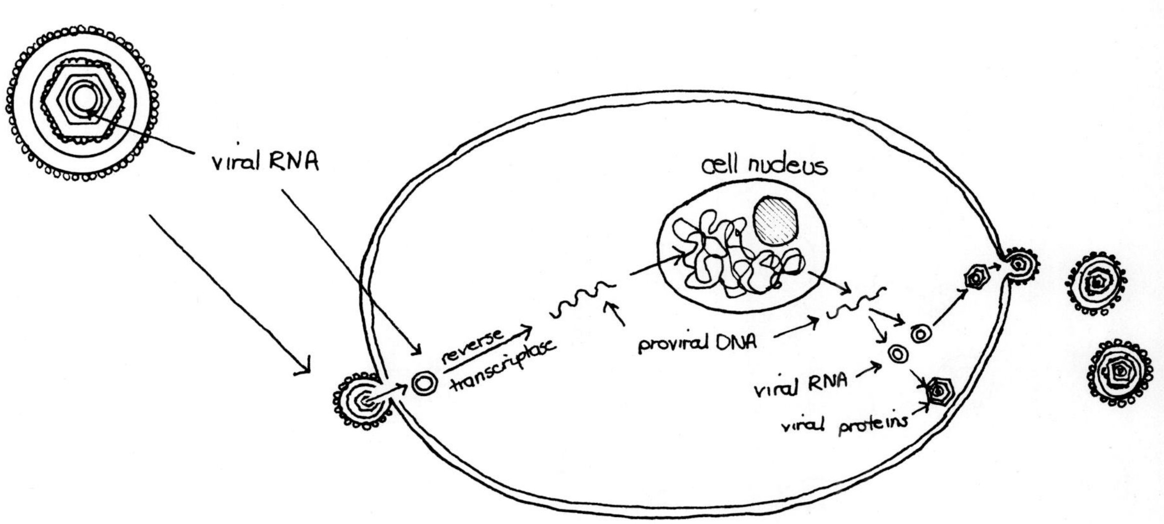

More often, the proviral DNA
does almost nothing for many years
until it suddenly is "activated" or "turns on."
No one knows what causes this to happen,
but doctors think it might be
another infection by another virus.
That would "turn on" the whole immune system,
especially T-cells.
Whatever causes the proviral DNA to turn on,
the result is the same.
The infected helper T-cell becomes a virus factory.
New HIVs are made,
and the helper T-cell is killed.
When lots of helper T-cells have been killed,
what happens is a T-cell immunodeficiency.
The person starts to get
all kinds of infections,
and these infections last longer
and are more serious than they would be otherwise.

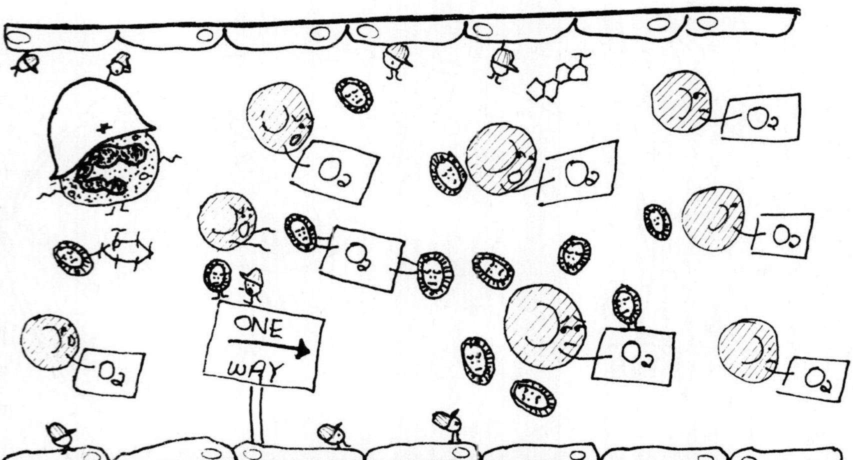

The rest of the cells in the immune system
can't do their work right, either.
This is partly because they don't have
the help and guidance of enough helper T-cells.
And, it's partly because of something else:
HIV can infect these other cells, too.
HIV can infect B-cells.
HIV can infect phagocytes, such as macrophages.
HIV doesn't kill these cells.
It just makes them sick,
and they can't do their jobs well.
HIV can infect all these cells
because they all have the CD-4 antigen
on their surfaces,
and the CD-4 antigen
is how HIV gets into cells.

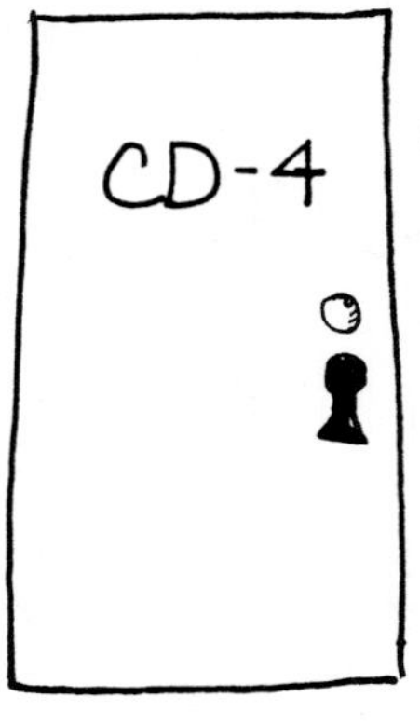

HIV causes immunodeficiency
many different ways.
The most important way is by
infecting helper T-cells,
making them into virus factories
and even killing them.
This would be enough to cause
a serious immune deficiency.
But because HIV can also infect
most of the other kinds of cells in the immune system,
making them sick or even killing them,
it can cause many kinds of immunodeficiencies
all at once.

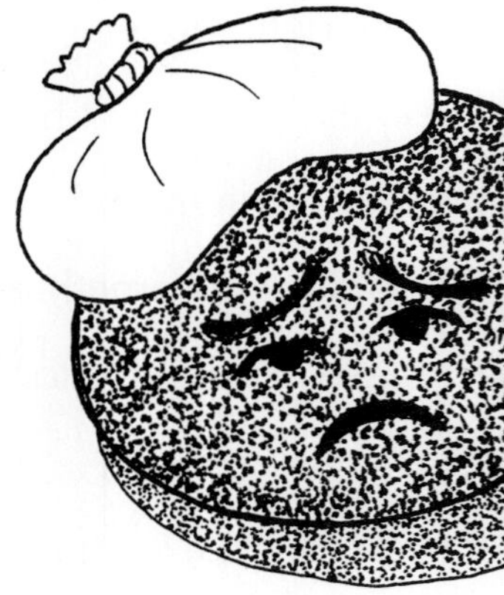

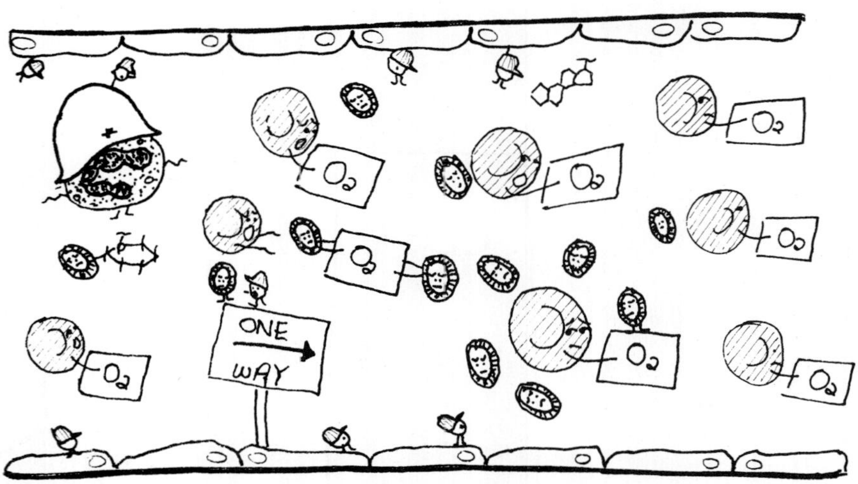

How Do Children Catch HIV?

All germs that like to infect people,
not just HIV,
have to figure out a way to get from
one person to another.
Germs have lots of ways of doing this.
A very popular way that a lot of germs use
is to make us sneeze and cough.
That's because when we sneeze or cough
we spray germs all over the room,
and other people breathe them in.
(This is why you should always cover
your mouth and nose when you sneeze or cough.)
Another popular way
is by hiding in dirt or dirty water
and getting onto things people eat or drink,
or just onto people's hands
and then, maybe, into their mouths.
(This is why it's important
to wash your hands often,
and to wash fresh fruits and vegetables,
in good, clean water.)

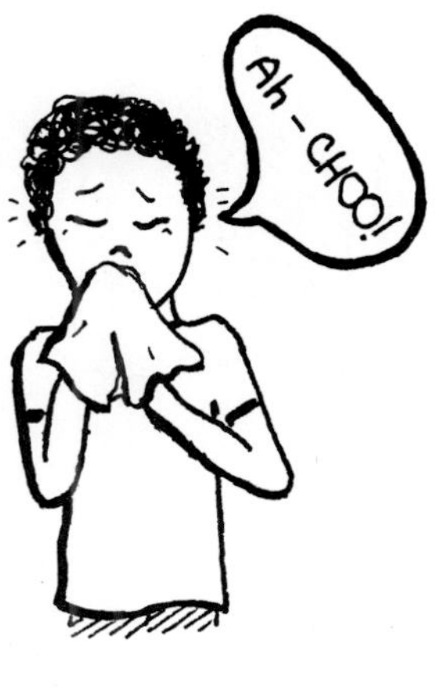

Other germs use other ways.
For instance, some germs use bugs that bite people,
such as mosquitoes, ticks or flies,
to get from one person to another.
One kind of germ uses snails.
Another uses dogs.
Some ride around on birds and animals.
Some hide inside foods like meats and raw milk.
Some really strong germs
just live in the ground
hoping someone with a cut foot
will step on them.
The germs that use these kinds of ways
are all pretty strong.
They have to be able to stay alive,
sometimes for a long time,
outside the human body.

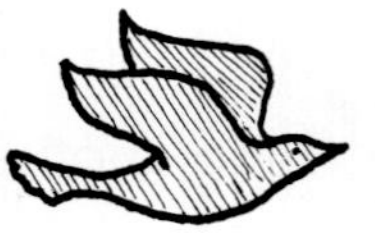

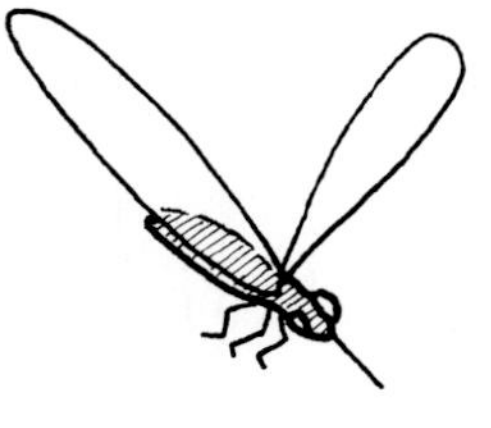

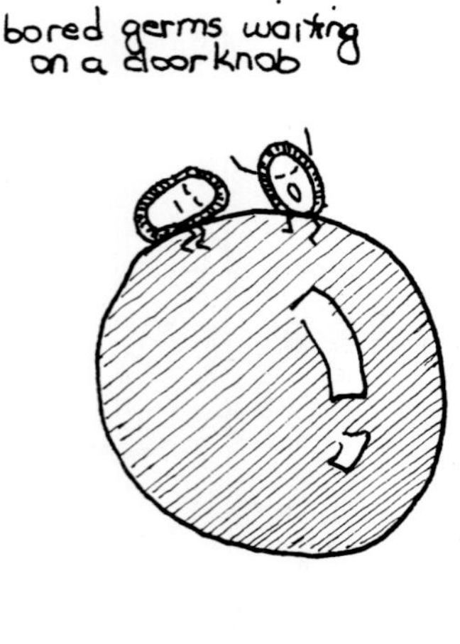

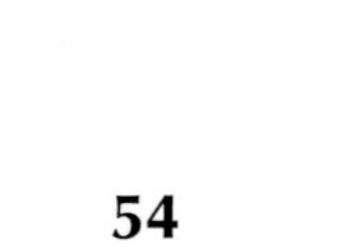

Not all germs that infect people
are strong enough to stay alive
outside a person's body
long enough to infect anyone else.
HIV is one of these weak germs.
HIV can only live
inside people's bodies.
The only way HIV can go
from one person to another
is when something from the *inside*
of an infected person's body
is put *inside* someone else's body,
carrying HIV along with it.
So, *you* didn't catch HIV
because someone sneezed or coughed
or forgot to wash their hands.
You didn't get it by eating bad food,
or from touching anything or anyone,
or being bitten by a bug.
And *no one else will ever catch HIV from you*
in any of these ways.

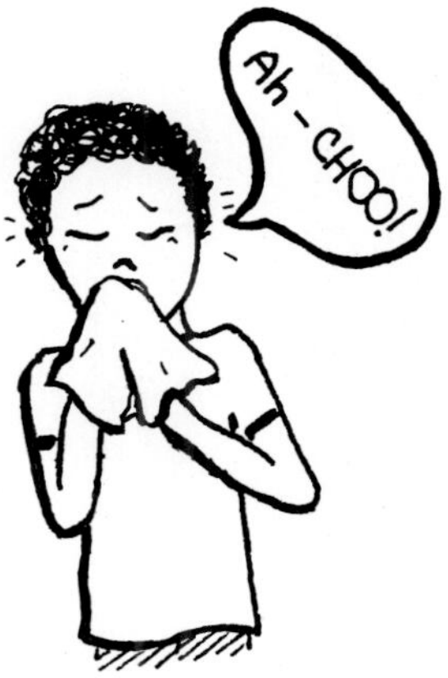

You caught HIV

because something from the inside

of an infected person's body

got into your body,

bringing HIV with it.

But how can this happen?

How can part of the *inside* of one person's body

get into another person's body?

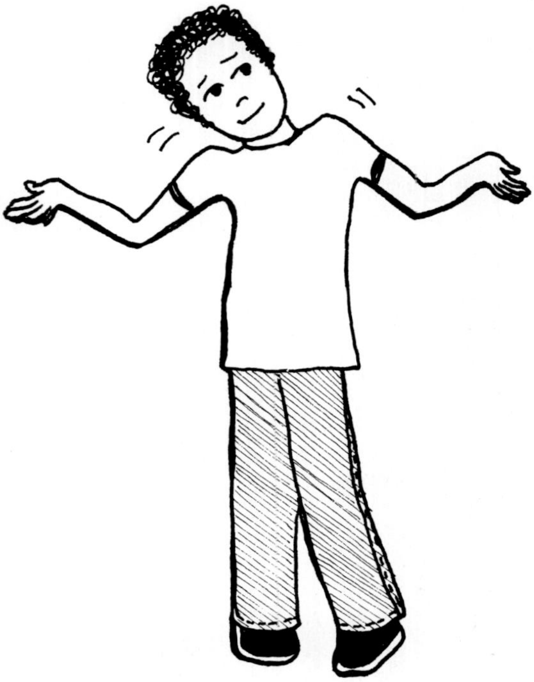

Well, blood is a part of the inside
of everyone's body.
And you already know that HIV infects
a lot of the cells that live in the blood.
So it would make sense
that if blood from an infected person
got put into the blood vessels of another person,
the second person could also get infected
with HIV.
It makes sense,
and it is one of the most common ways
that HIV is spread
from one person to another.

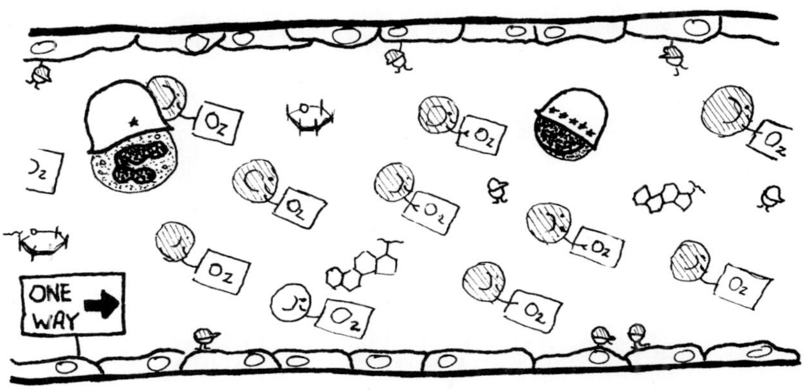

Another way that a part of one person's body
can get inside another person's body
is when two people have sex.
Sex is something that grownups do
to show their love for each other
by having their bodies very close together.
Sex is also how your father's sperm
got together with your mother's egg
to make the cell that would become you.
When two grownups get this close,
it is possible for one of them to give the other one
a germ like HIV by accident.
You'll probably have a lot of questions about sex
as you get older.
There are some very good books about it
listed at the back of this book.

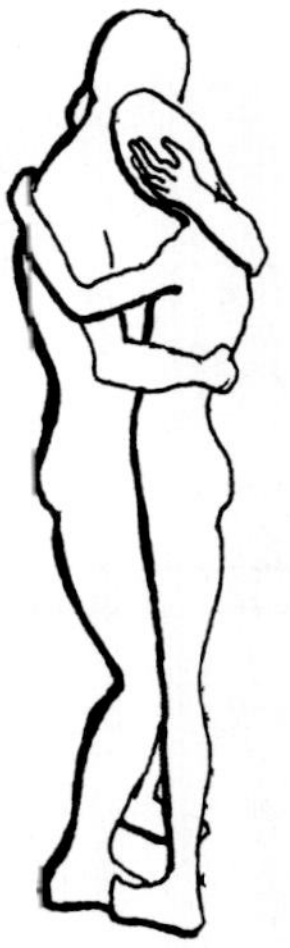

Almost all children who have HIV
got it because someone else's infected blood
was put into their bodies.
This has happened in a number of ways.

One way was by being given a blood transfusion
that accidentally had HIV in it.

Another way was by being given blood products
that accidentally had HIV in them.
(Blood products are medicines made out of things in plasma.
They are used to help people whose plasma
is missing these things,
such as people with a disease called hemophilia.)

Now that doctors know about HIV,
all blood used in blood transfusions
or to make blood products
is tested to be sure there is no HIV in it.

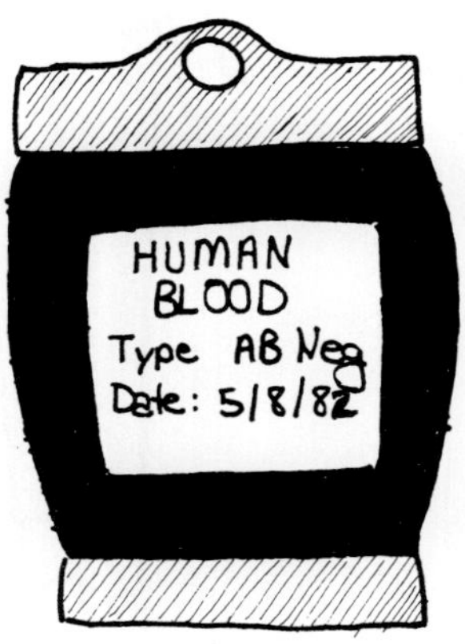

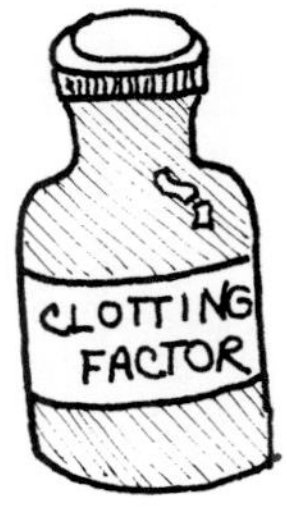

The most common way that children get HIV
by having someone else's blood get in their bodies
is by being born to a mother who has HIV.
When a baby grows inside its mother,
she shares some of the things in her blood
with her baby.
The baby needs her to do that.
This is how babies get oxygen and food
before they are able to breathe or eat.
This is how babies get antibodies
to protect them from getting sick
soon after they are born.
But, if the mother is infected with HIV,
or any other germ,
she can accidentally share her germs, too.

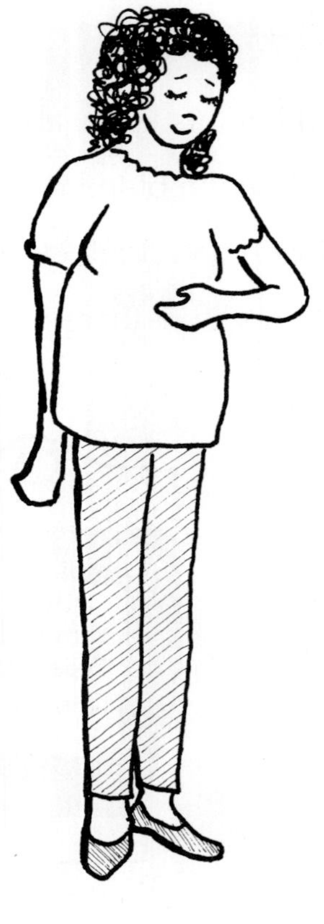

Every person who is now infected with HIV,
whether they are children or grownups,
caught it from another person
who caught it from still another person.
Now that blood can be tested
to see if it has HIV in it,
children don't have to be scared about getting HIV
from either blood transfusions
or from using blood products.
HIV is almost never spread by these ways anymore.
Doctors are also trying hard to find ways
to prevent mothers who have HIV
from accidentally giving it to their babies.
Doctors are also trying
to make vaccines (see pages 162-163)
that will protect people who don't have HIV
from getting it,
and protect people who do have HIV
from getting sick because of it.

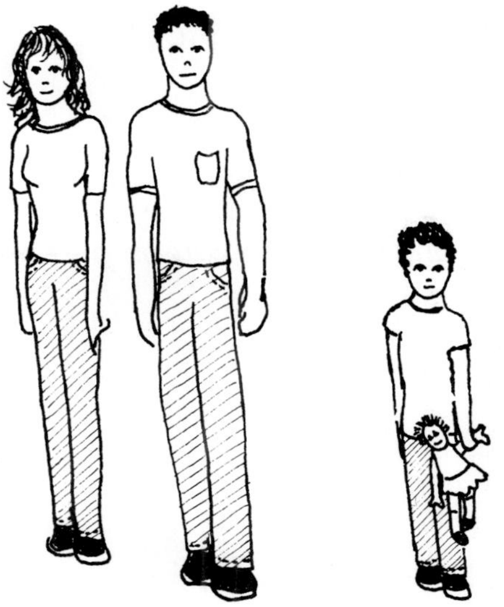

However you got HIV,
you need to know that it wasn't your fault.
Maybe you're afraid that something you did
might have caused it.
Maybe you think
that your HIV infection is a punishment for something.
That if you or someone else is "bad,"
you might get sicker.
These things are just not true.

You may also wonder
if someone wanted you to have HIV
and figured out a way to give it to you.
You may want to blame and punish that person.
But that wouldn't be fair.
No one wanted you to have HIV.

So, it's very important that you
always remember two things:

> *It is not your fault that you have HIV.*
> *No one gave it to you on purpose.*

How Doctors Diagnose HIV

Your body is a wonderful thing,
but it is not perfect.
Sometimes something goes wrong.
It can be hurt on the outside.
You might fall down and skin your knee.
When something goes wrong on the outside of you,
you know a lot about it.
You can see it and touch it.
Your doctor can see it and touch it, too.
Just by looking at you, your doctor will know
if you are getting better.

Things can go wrong on your inside, too.
You can't see it or touch it,
but it's wrong just the same.
Only it's harder to understand.
It's harder for your doctor, too.
But doctors have special ways
to learn what's going on inside of you.
Many of these ways were used to find out
if you had HIV.

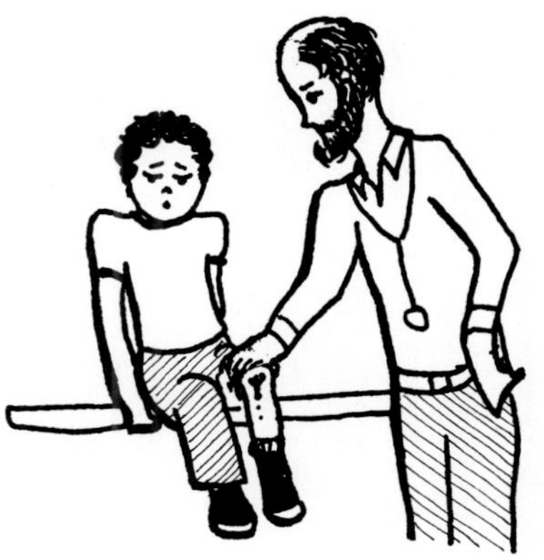

You and the grownups who live with you
know more about you and how you feel
than anyone else.
So, one of the best ways
for doctors to learn about what you have
is to ask a lot of questions
of you and your parents or caretaker,
and to listen carefully to your answers.
This is called "taking a history."
In school, history means learning about the past.
When a doctor takes your history,
he or she is learning about *your* past.
The doctor will want to know all about you
before and after you were born.
The most important thing to the doctor
at that moment
is the story of your life!

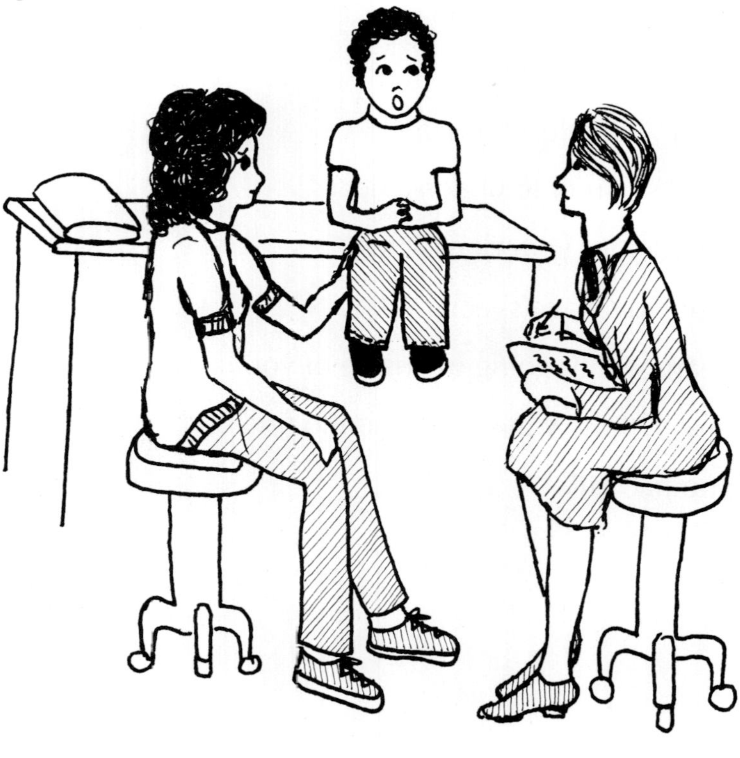

The doctor will especially want to know
about any health problems you have had
and about how you are feeling now.
Most diseases have symptoms.
Symptoms are the things *you* feel or notice
that aren't right.
Symptoms are the reasons that you go to the doctor.
The doctor will ask you questions about your symptoms.
If you have symptoms of HIV infection,
what are they?
The most common symptoms of HIV infection in children are:

1. getting sick a lot
2. fevers and night sweats
3. swollen glands in your neck
4. big lymph nodes
5. rashes
6. diarrhea
7. a cough that won't go away
8. weight loss
9. not growing as fast as other kids
10. having trouble thinking, talking, or walking
11. feeling tired all the time
12. a big, swollen tummy

Every disease has signs.

Signs are what the *doctor* finds

when he or she is examining you.

They tell your doctor that something isn't right.

If you had signs of HIV infection,

do you remember what they were?

The most common signs of HIV infection in children are:

1. big lymph nodes
2. big spleen and liver
3. fever
4. a white tongue and throat (thrush)
5. swollen glands in your neck
6. cough
7. pale skin and gums
8. yellow skin and eyeballs
9. ear, throat, skin, or other infections
10. being small for your age
11. being kind of sleepy or weak and floppy
12. having a hard time paying attention

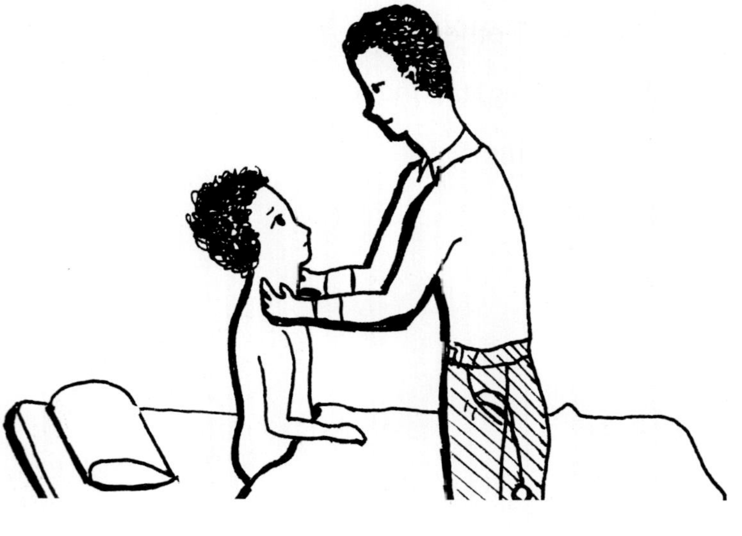

The reason the doctor has to ask so many questions
and examine you all over
is because HIV infection is tricky.
Not everyone whose history
includes things that make it possible to have HIV
turns out to have it.
Sometimes people have nothing in their history
that would make a doctor think of HIV infection,
yet, they are infected.
Many people who are infected with HIV
have no signs or symptoms at all
(this is called "asymptomatic HIV infection").
Also, there are other diseases besides HIV
that can cause these signs and symptoms.
Most children have fevers or big lymph nodes
at one time or another.
And lots of kids get infections.
All of this can make it hard for the doctor
to figure out what is wrong, at first.
So, the doctor will want to do one more thing:
look at your blood
and have it tested for HIV.

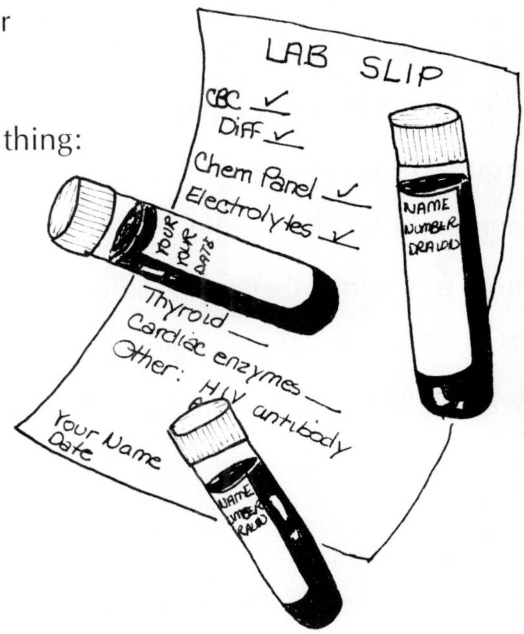

Blood Tests

For doctors to look at and test your blood
they have to get a little of it from you.
This can be done many ways.
The easiest way is just to make a little prick
in one of your fingers.
Another way is to put a needle
into one of your blood vessels.
These kinds of blood tests hurt, but not very much,
and they don't take very long.

If you have a central line (see pages 229-235),
it can be used to get blood for testing.

The person who takes your blood for the test
will probably wear thin latex gloves.
These gloves are to prevent any germs
that are on his or her hands
from getting onto or into you—
and to protect him or her
from any germs that might be in your blood.
They always wear these gloves
when getting blood from people—not just you.

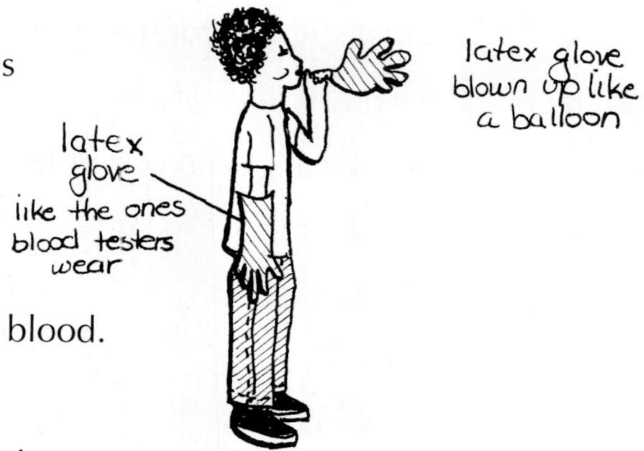
latex glove like the ones blood testers wear
latex glove blown up like a balloon

Once your doctor has some of your blood
a lot of things will happen to it.
We thought you'd like to know what they are.
One part of your blood will be used
for HIV tests.
Another part will be looked at
and the different kinds of cells in it
will be counted.
Still another part will be given
what is called a chemistry test.
You will learn all about these different tests
in this section.

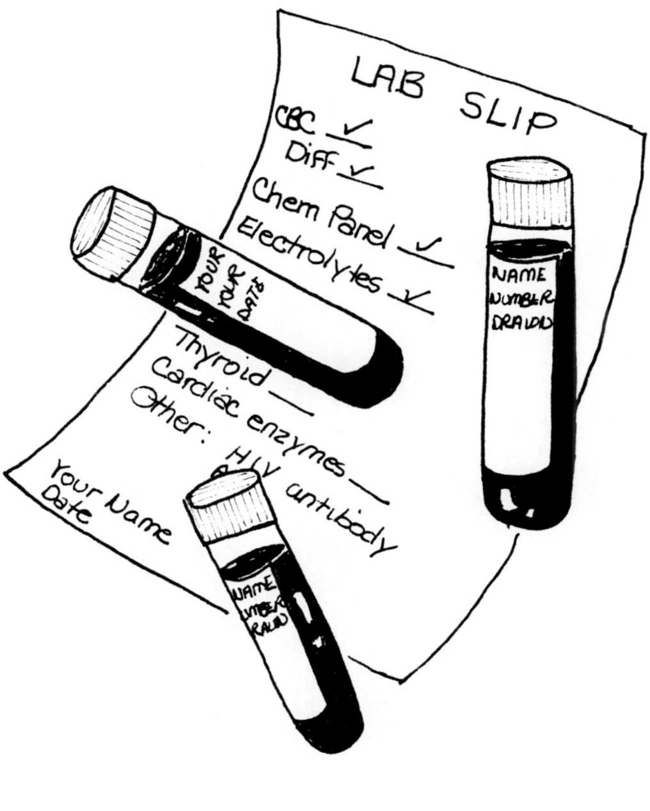

HIV Antibody Tests

You already know what antibody is:
the stuff that B-cells make
that sticks to germ antigens.
HIV has antigens like any other germ,
so when it got into your body,
your immune system tried to destroy it.
One of the ways that it tried
was by having your B-cells turn into plasma cells
and make antibody.
There are two tests
that look for antibody against HIV.
One is called the ELISA test.
The other is called the Western Blot test.
When these tests are both "positive,"
it means that antibody against HIV
has been found in your blood.

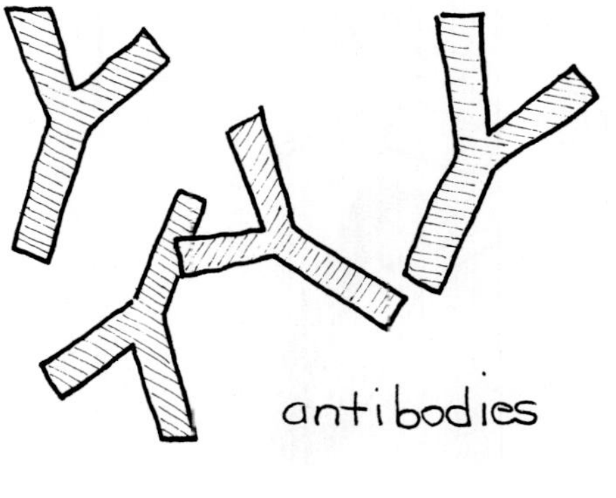

HIV Antigen Tests

You already know what antigens are.
They are the nametags on our cells
that tell what kind of cells they are
and who they belong to.
They are also the nametags on germs
that tell what kind of germs they are.
Viruses use their antigens like keys
to unlock the doors into cells.
HIV has antigens like any virus.
These have funny names,
like p18, p25, gp41 and gp120.
Doctors can make antibody
that will stick to any one of these antigens.
By mixing this antibody with your blood
doctors can sometimes tell
if you are infected with HIV
even if you don't have any antibody to HIV.

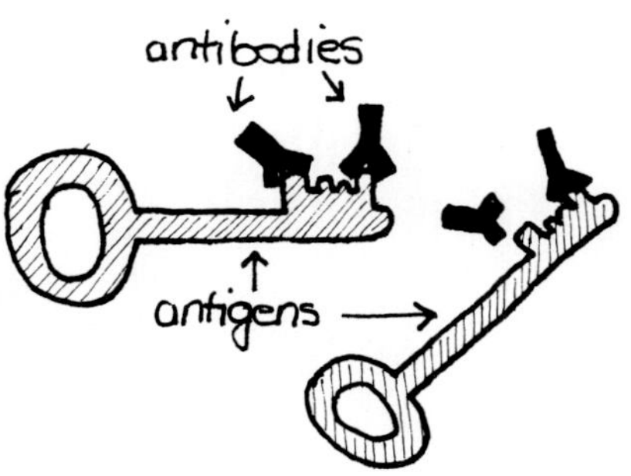

HIV Cultures

Most germs that grow inside a person's body
can also be grown outside it.
This is done by putting a tiny drop of blood
(or a tiny drop of something else from your body)
in something called a "growth medium."
A growth medium is just a little world
full of the things the germ they're looking for
needs to have to grow.
For *you,* the perfect growth medium
is your home and the people you love, good food and water,
and warm clothes when it's cold.
A growth medium for germs looks very different from yours—
for example, it's a lot smaller—
but it's just as warm and cozy to a germ.
Like all germs, HIV can be grown outside the body.
This isn't done very often,
but because you may need blood or other cultures done
to find HIV or other germs,
we thought you should know what they are.
Ask your doctor to show you a growth medium sometime.
(*You* won't want to live there!)

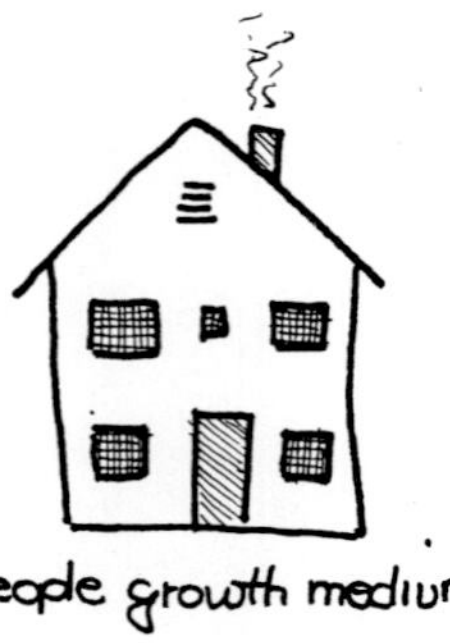

people growth medium

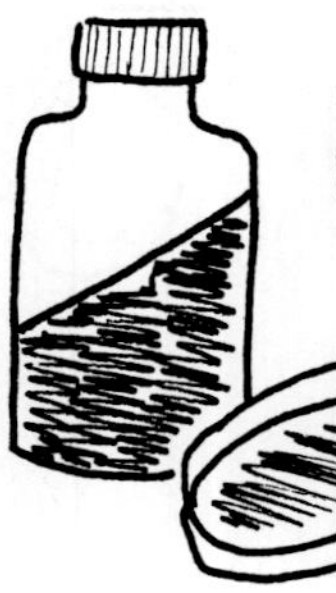

germ
growth
medium

HIV PCR Tests

There is one more test for HIV
that you might have or hear about.
That is the PCR test.
This is a short way of saying,
"polymerase chain reaction."
What this test does is look for
loose pieces of the HIV RNA plan,
or the proviral DNA that is made from it.
These pieces, or genes, have funny names
like "gag," "pol" and "env."
Like the HIV antigen tests or HIV cultures,
the PCR test looks for HIV itself
(or pieces of it),
so it can tell if you have HIV
even if your immune system
hasn't made antibodies to HIV.
The PCR test may be the best one for doctors to use
to tell if babies who are born to mothers with HIV
are infected with HIV themselves.

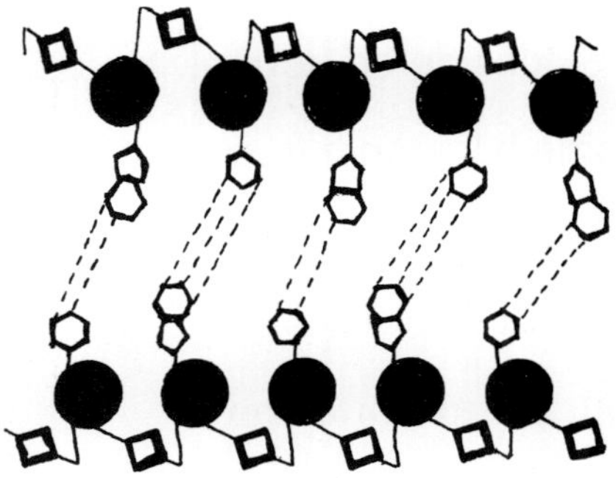

Blood Counts

Another thing doctors will do with your blood
is to look at it.
A drop of your blood will be put
on a thin piece of glass called a "slide,"
and be spread out until it's very thin.
Then the doctor will look at it
through a microscope—
a special instrument that makes tiny things
look very, very big.
The doctor wants to know if all the cells
that should be there, are there.
Blood is very pretty
when you look at it through a microscope.
Ask your doctor to show it to you sometime.
You'll be amazed.

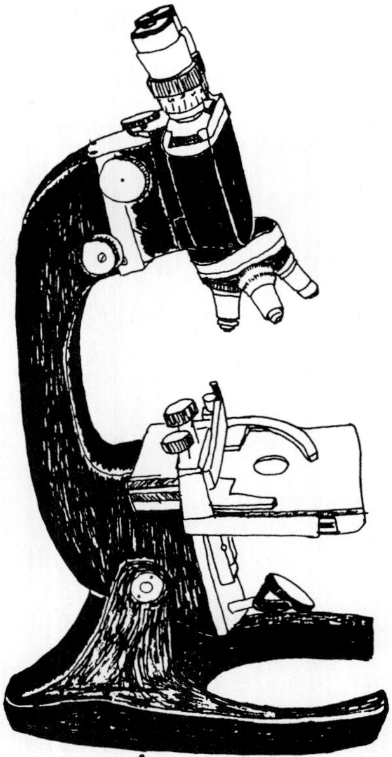

All your different kinds of cells
will be counted, too, by a person or a machine.
When your blood cells have been counted,
your numbers will be compared
with the numbers that are considered normal.
Your blood count will come back on a form
kind of like the one on the next page,
or else on a computer printout.
(You may want to ask your doctor for a copy
of the form used at your treatment center.)

PATIENT ______________________ CHG. ______________

DOCTOR ______________________ DATE ______________

HEMATOLOGY

	Complete blood count			Differential			Bleeding	
X	Hemoglobin	gms		Segmented	%		Ven. Coag. Time	
	Hematocrit			Band	%		Cap. Coag. Time	
	Sed. Rate mm/hr.						Prothrombin Time	
X	WBC			Eosinophiles	%		Control	sec.
X	RBC millions			Basophiles	%		Patient Time	sec.
	MCHC		X	Lymphocytes	%		Ratio $(\frac{PT}{C})$ =	
	MCH			Monocytes	%		Therapeutic Range 1.5-1.8	
	MCV						PTT	
	Color Index						Norm Less Than 40 sec.	
	Reticulocytes		RBC Morphology:					
X	Platelets							
	Mono Spot							
	R. F. Latex							

There are a lot of words on here.

These are the important ones if you have HIV.

The number next to "WBC" is your white blood cell count.

Normal is about 4 to 11.

The number next to "RBC" is your red blood cell count.

Normal is about 4 to 5.

The number next to "Hemoglobin" (also called "HGB")

tells how well your RBCs are doing

at their job of carrying oxygen to your other cells.

Normal is about 11 to 14 for children.

The number next to "Platelets" is your platelet count.

Normal is about 140 to 400.

The number next to "Lymphoctyes"

is used to figure out how many lymphocytes you have.

None of these numbers tell your doctor
if you have HIV or not.
Only HIV tests can do that.
But these numbers tell your doctor
things about how well you're doing.
HIV can cause you to have
low RBC or HBG counts (anemia),
low platelet counts (thrombocytopenia),
and low lymphocyte counts (lymphopenia).
Some medicines you might take
to help you get better from HIV itself,
or from the infections you can get,
can make those counts low
and can also make your WBC counts low (leukopenia).
In fact, if you have HIV,
low counts will be normal for you.
Your doctor will try to make sure that
these counts never get low enough to cause you trouble.
When you have HIV,
blood counts are an important part of your life.

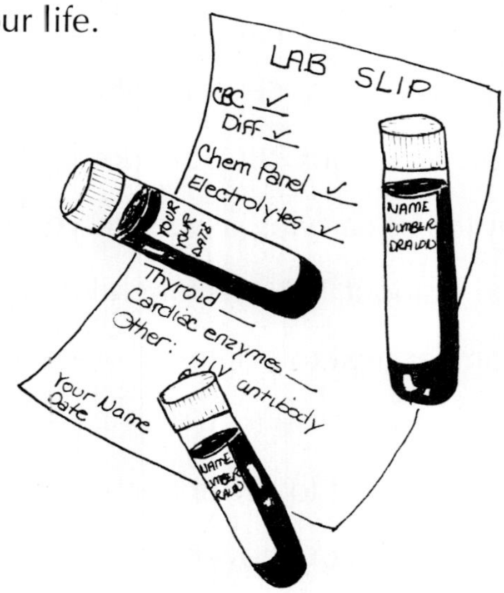

Lymphoctye Counts

While your regular blood count
tells doctors about how many lymphocytes you have,
it doesn't tell anything
about the different kinds of lymphocytes.
In HIV, it's important to know this.
So, doctors have ways
to tell different kinds of lymphocytes apart.
They do this by making antibodies
to the special antigens on lymphocytes
such as the CD-4 antigen.
They stick shiny stuff on these antibodies
so that when they look at your lymphocytes
through a microscope,
the ones they want to count will light up
like Christmas trees.
That makes them very easy to count
(and really nice to look at).

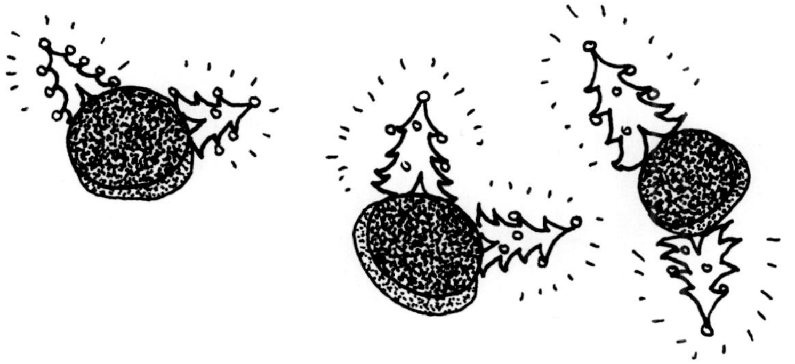

There are two types of lymphocytes
your doctors will be most interested in counting.
One is your helper T-cells, or T4 cells.
These are the ones with the CD-4 antigen,
the cells that HIV infects.
A normal T4 count is more than 1000 for most people,
and more than 3000 for babies.
In HIV, it is often lower.
The other type of lymphocyte your doctors like to count
is your suppressor T-cells, or T8 cells.
HIV does not infect T8 cells.
Usually, the T8 count is lower than the T4 count.
In HIV, it often isn't.
By counting your T4 cells,
and by comparing your T4 count with your T8 count,
your doctor can figure out
how much trouble your immunodeficiency
may be giving you.
Your doctor might give you medicines
to prevent dangerous infections
if your T4 count gets too low.
Lymphocyte counts really help
your doctor take care of you.

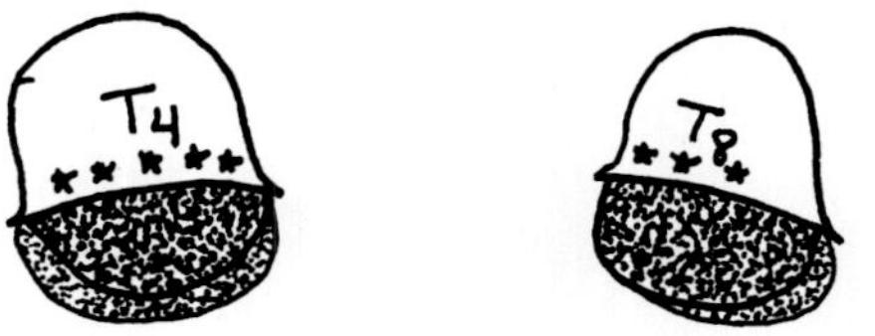

Blood Chemistry Tests

HIV is mainly a problem of the immune system,
but it can affect other organ systems, too.
Some organs in these other organ systems
make chemical things that end up in your blood.
By looking for these chemicals,
doctors can learn how these organs are doing.
HIV can affect your liver,
so doctors will measure things your liver makes,
such as LDH,
to see how your liver is doing.

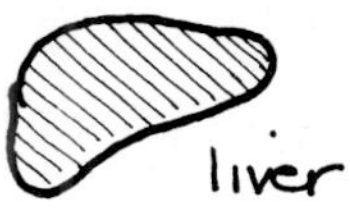

HIV can affect your kidneys,
so doctors will measure things your kidney makes,
like BUN and creatinine,
to see how your kidneys are doing.

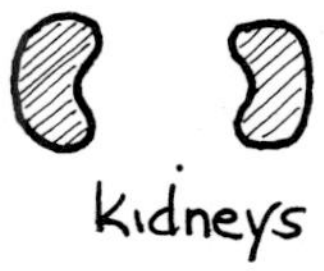

HIV can cause your B-cells
to make all sorts of extra antibody,
so doctors will measure
the amount of antibody in your blood,
like IgG or gamma globulin,
to see how your B-cells are doing.

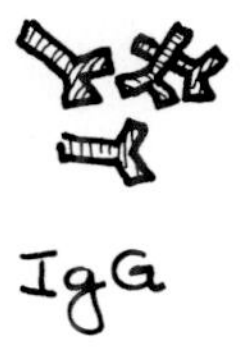

Blood tests tell what's happening
everywhere in your body,
not just in your blood.

Now that you and your doctor know
that you have HIV,
blood tests are going to be
a regular thing for you.
There isn't a child in the world—
or even a grownup—
who likes having blood tests
so you probably won't like it either.
We thought it would help, though,
if you knew just how much
your doctors can learn about you
and how to take care of you better
by testing just a little bit of your blood.
And they really only need a little bit
to do all these tests.

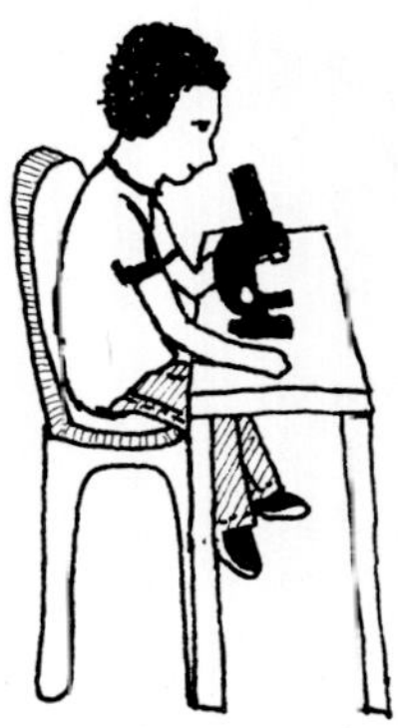

You—looking at your very own blood through a microscope. It's pretty!

Stages of HIV Infection

Every disease or infection has stages,
or beginnings, middles and ends.
Each stage has its own name or names.

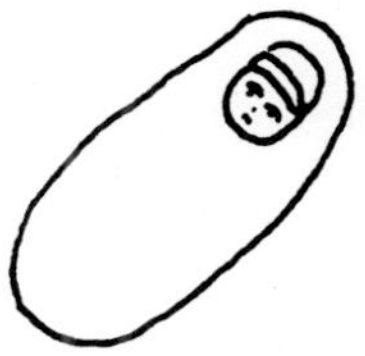

One stage of HIV infection in babies
is called "Indeterminate HIV Infection."
That means, the baby's mother has HIV
and the baby has antibodies to HIV—
but no one can figure out for sure
if the baby itself has HIV.

Another stage of HIV infection in both kids and grownups
is called "Asymptomatic HIV Infection."
This is when a person is known to have HIV,
but it hasn't made him or her sick yet.
This is kind of the beginning stage of HIV,
and it can last for a short time
or for many, many years.

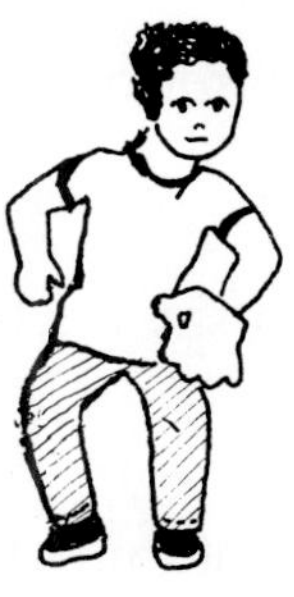

The next stage of HIV infection
is called "Symptomatic HIV Infection."
This is when HIV has hurt the immune system enough
to cause immunodeficiency,
and the person starts to have other infections
or complications of HIV (see pages 94-121).
This is the middle stage of HIV, and it can last for many years.

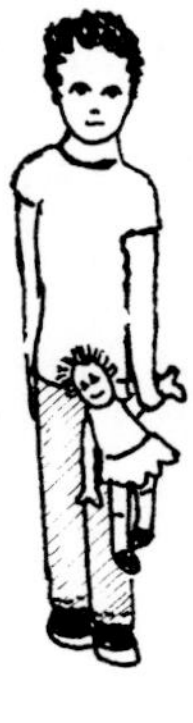

Symptomatic HIV infection has other names.
The one most people have heard is AIDS,
which is short for "**A**cquired **I**mmuno**d**eficiency **S**yndrome."
When children have AIDS,
it is sometimes called PAIDS,
which is short for "**P**ediatric AIDS."

Other names for symptomatic HIV infection are:
ARC (which is short for "**A**IDS-**R**elated **C**omplex");
PGL (which is short for
"**P**ersistent **G**eneralized **L**ymphadenopathy"); and
LAS (which is short for "**L**ymph**a**denopathy **S**yndrome").

The terms AIDS and PAIDS are used
to talk about children with symptomatic HIV infection.
The other terms are only used
to talk about grownups with symptomatic HIV infection,
so we won't say anything more about them in this book.

The important thing to remember
is that "symptomatic HIV infection," AIDS, and PAIDS
all mean the same thing:
the middle stage of HIV infection.

The ending, or last stage, of any disease
is always one of two things:
either the disease goes away and the person is cured
or the disease takes the person's life.
Because there is as yet no cure for HIV,
no one has ever gotten better from it.
But that doesn't necessarily mean
that HIV will take your life.
There are lots of diseases—
such as diabetes and cancer—
that used to take the lives of many children
and now don't.
Doctors have learned how to *treat* these diseases,
even if they don't know how to *cure* some of them.
So the people with the diseases just live with them—
the way they live with the color of their eyes—
as a part of themselves that they must accept
because they can't really change it.
HIV is a disease like diabetes,
one that can't be cured yet,
but one that doctors are getting better at controlling.
At this time, this is what the treatment of HIV
is all about.

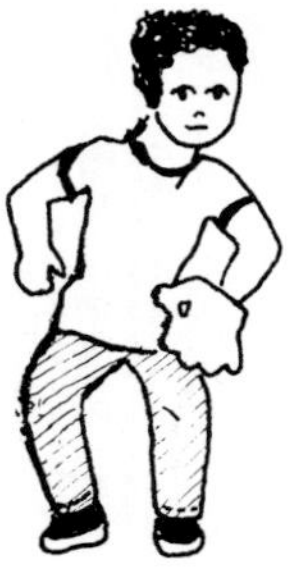

How Doctors Treat HIV

Now that you know you have HIV,
what can be done to make you better?
Not long ago, there was nothing that could be done.
That's because until 1983 no one, including doctors,
even knew that HIV existed.
But in the last few years, doctors and scientists
have found medicines that make life difficult for HIV.
This is called "antiviral therapy."
They have also found ways
to help the immune system work better.
These are called "immune boosters."
And, doctors are getting better
at treating the many complications of HIV.
This is called "supportive therapy."
Most children with HIV get all three kinds of therapy.
The treatment that you will get
will be based on the best one that's been found so far.
But experiments with new medicines
and combinations of medicines
are going on all the time
to find even better treatments.

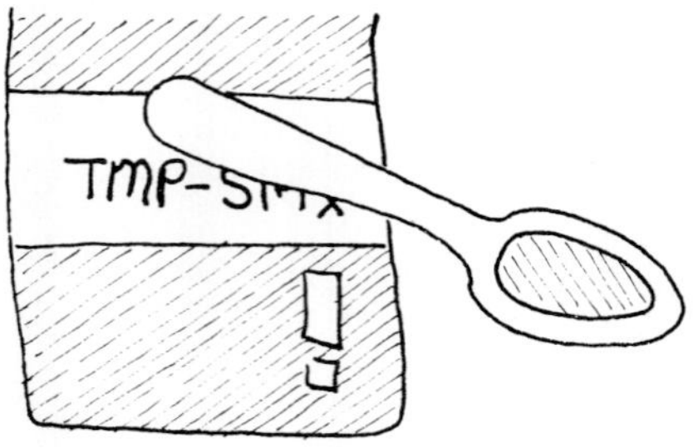

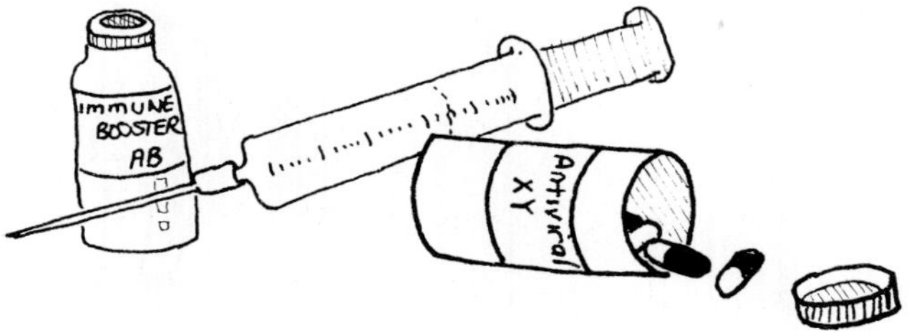

You may be asked to try a new medicine
as part of an experimental treatment program.
These programs are usually called protocols.
If you are "on study" or "on a protocol,"
this means that you will get exactly the same treatment
everyone else on that protocol will get—
no matter where you and they live.
If you decide to be in an experimental program,
you will get the best of the proven medicines
and the best of the new medicines.
If you decide not to be in an experimental program,
you can still have the best of the proven medicines.

Or, *you* may want to try a new medicine,
but your doctor may not be part of an experimental program.
If your doctor isn't, and you want to try a new medicine,
ask your doctor to help you get into a center
where experimental medicines are being tried.
You and your doctor can find out about these programs
by calling the clinical trials information services of the
National Institute of Allergy and Infectious Diseases,
1-800-TRIALS-A;
and the Pediatric Branch of the National Cancer Institute,
1-301-496-4256 (call collect).
Being part of a program to find
new and better treatments for HIV
is one way you may help yourself
and help other people, too.

Antiviral Therapy

Antiviral therapy means medicines
that either kill or cripple HIV.
You know so much about HIV now
that you can probably figure out
ways this could be done.
The ways that scientists and doctors are trying are:

1. making it hard for HIV to get into cells
2. making it hard for the viral RNA to make proviral DNA
3. making it hard for the proviral DNA to join with the cell's DNA
4. making it hard for the proviral DNA to turn the cell into a virus factory
5. making it hard for the almost-finished viruses to get out of the infected cell

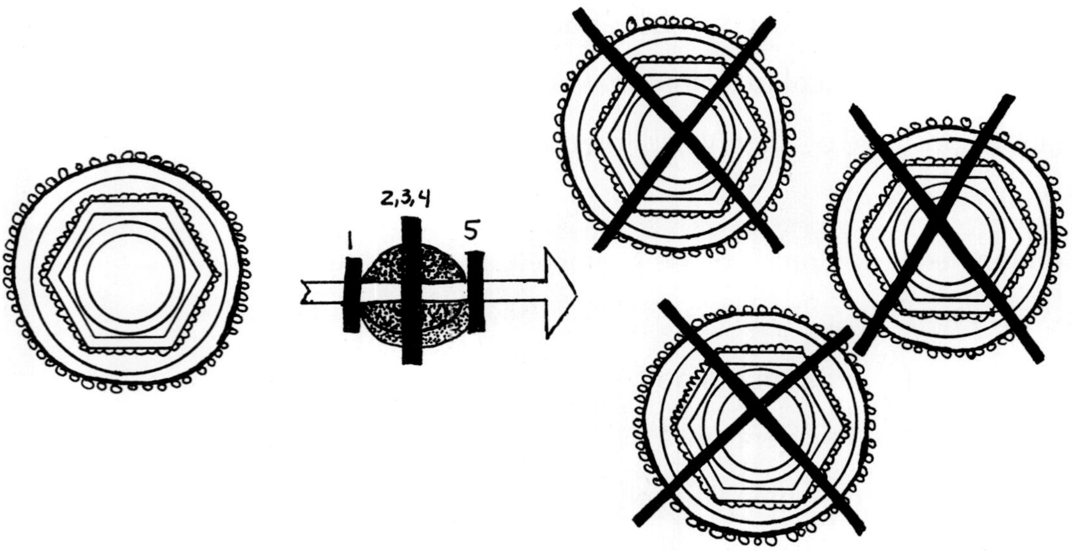

Scientists and doctors are trying all these ways.
They have had the best luck so far
with the second way.
There are a number of medicines
that inhibit, or really slow down,
reverse transcriptase—
the put-together kind of enzyme
HIV uses to make proviral DNA
from its own RNA plan.
AZT, or Retrovir, is the one that's been used longest,
and it has worked very well for lots of people,
including children.
There are other medicines that work this way.
Of these, the one that has been found to work best
is ddI,
and it is now being tried in children.
These kinds of medicines don't cure HIV,
but they can slow it down.
More information about all the antiviral medicines
now being used or tested
can be found in the Special Section on Treatment
at the back of the book.

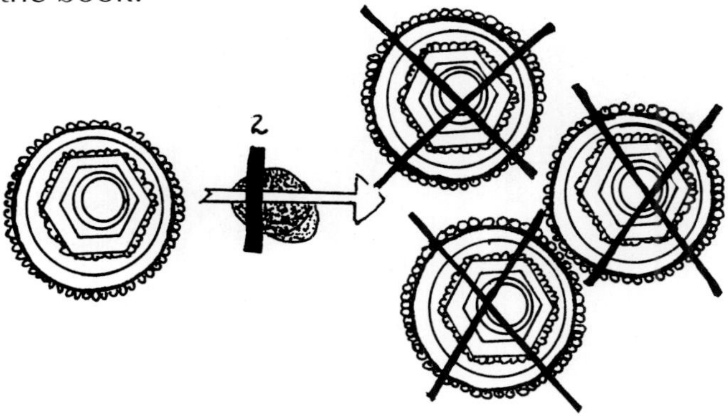

Doctors are now also trying the first way,
trying to make life difficult for HIV
by making it harder for it to get into cells.
They are doing this by using
something called "soluble CD4."
CD-4, you remember, is the antigen on helper T-cells
that HIV uses to unlock the door into the cells.
Soluble CD4 is just a whole bunch of CD-4 antigens—
only they're not part of any cell.
They're just loose, floating around in the blood.
Doctors hope HIV won't be able to tell the difference
between CD-4 that is part of a cell
and CD-4 that isn't.
This could trick the HIV
into thinking it was getting somewhere
when it really wasn't,
and stop many of them from ever getting into new cells.
No one knows if this way will work yet,
but it is now being tried in adults and children.
Soluble CD4 won't cure HIV,
but it may slow it down.

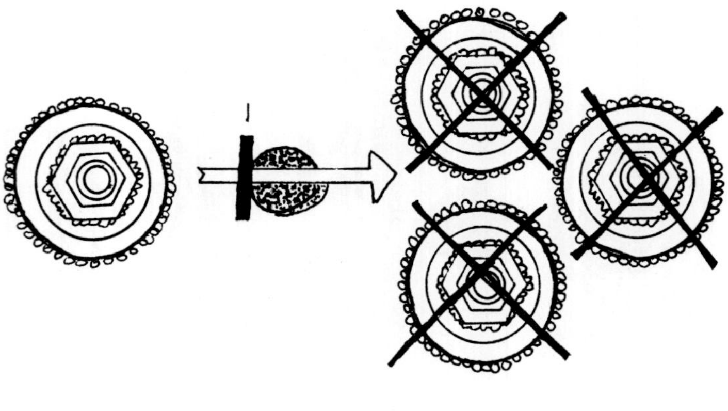

Immune Boosters

Immune boosters, which are also called
"immunomodulators" or "biologicals,"
are medicines that help your immune system
do its job of protecting you better.
The main kind of immune booster used in children
is IVIG.
IG is a short way of saying "immunoglobulins."
Immunoglobulins are just plain old antibodies.
If your immune system isn't making good antibodies,
your doctor may want to give you
antibodies from other people
to help protect you against common infections.

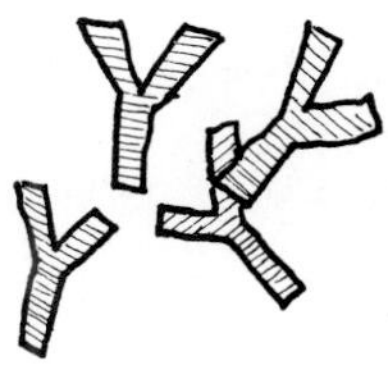

IV is a short way of saying "intravenous."
Intravenous means that something is put
right into a vein.
Getting a medicine—or anything else— "IV"
is kind of like getting a blood test,
except it takes longer
(but it usually doesn't hurt more).
So, IVIG just means antibodies
that you get intravenously.
Other kinds of immune boosters
are discussed at the back of the book.

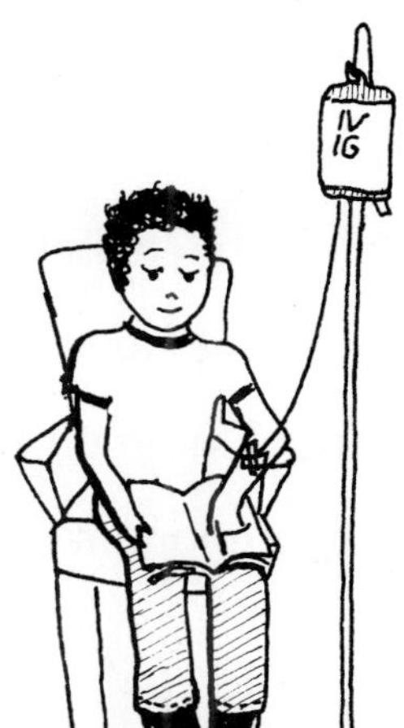

Supportive Therapy

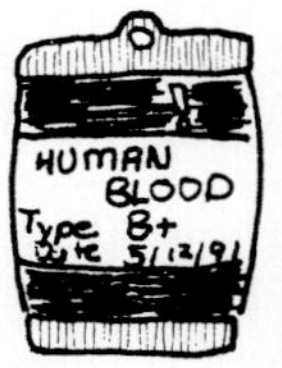

Supportive therapy means
medicines and other things
that will help you feel better
even though they have nothing to do
with slowing down or getting rid of HIV itself,
or with helping your immune system.
HIV can cause the people it infects
to have lots of different kinds of problems.

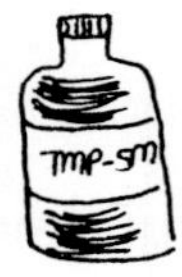

Supportive therapy is used
to help solve these other problems
and keep you as well as possible
while the search for better treatments for HIV goes on.
All through the rest of the book
you will learn about different kinds of problems
people with HIV can have,
and the kinds of supportive therapies
your doctors and your treatment team—
including you and your parent or caretaker—
can use to help you feel better.

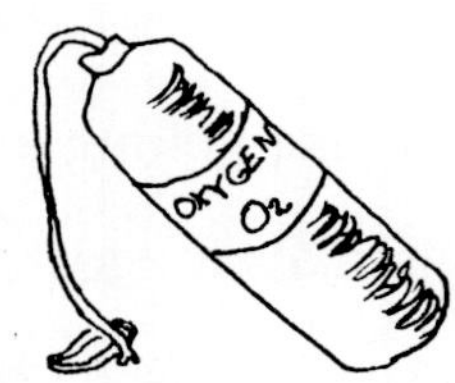

While supportive therapy can't cure HIV,
it can cure a lot of these other problems—
and that's really important for you.

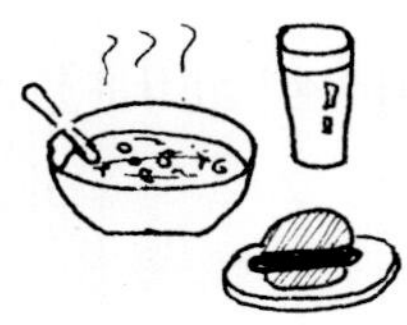

This page is for you and your doctors to use to write down your personal treatment plan.

My Treatment Plan

While treatment for HIV infection
is improving all the time,
there is still no cure.
That's why enjoying every healthy day
is very important.
If your HIV infection gets out of control,
it can take your life.
If your doctors feel your life is in danger,
they may want you to go to the hospital for a while
to get special treatment.
Hospitals aren't as nice as being at home,
but you'll have lots of friends there
and often a parent or caretaker can stay with you.
It's very important for you to know
that whatever happens
you won't be alone,
you will be loved,
and you will always be special.

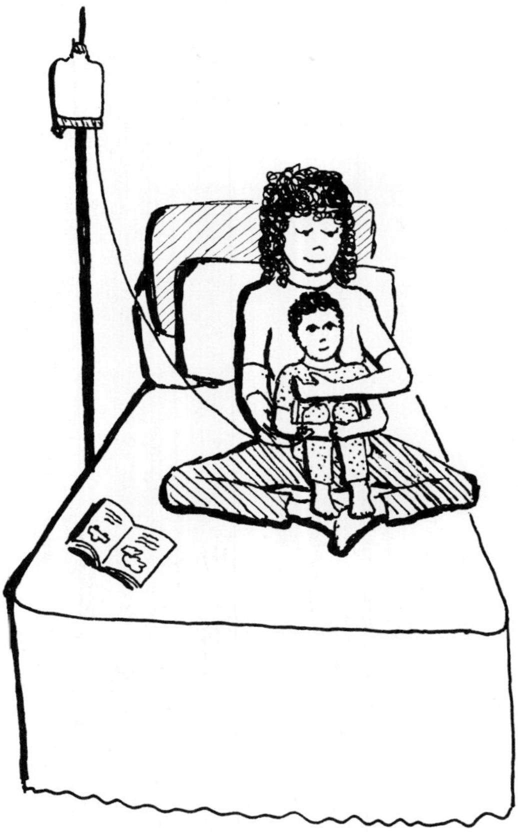

This is the last page of this section about treatment.
It is a good place to talk about forms of treatment
that most reputable doctors don't use
but that you might hear about
from friends, neighbors or relatives.
Whenever there is a disease that has no cure,
all sorts of people invent things they say will cure it.
These can be vitamins, special diets
or certain "medicines."
Some faith healers or spiritualists say they can cure HIV.
Most of these methods are not harmful
so it's OK to try them if you want to—
as long as you're also getting regular medical care.
If you want to try one of these treatments,
all we can do is ask
that you discuss it with your doctors.
You have a lot to gain from regular care.

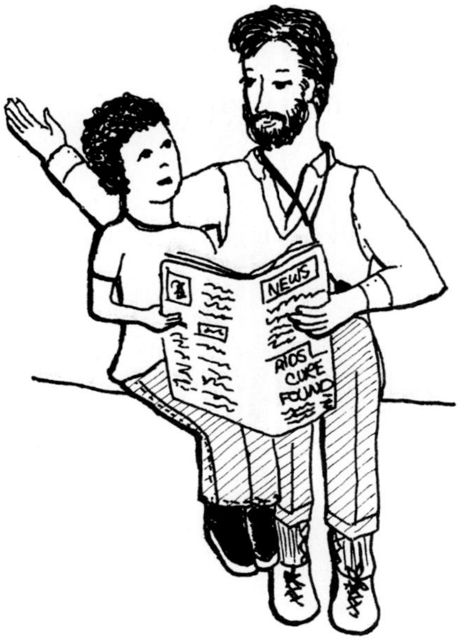

Complications of HIV

You know how important it is
that all of your cells and organs and systems
work right and work together.
So, it's easy to figure out that when
something goes wrong with one part of you,
all of you is affected.
In a city, if all the telephone lines fall down,
everybody is affected,
even though nothing is wrong with them.

With you, only some cells are infected with HIV,
yet your whole body is affected.
The other things that can be problems
are called complications.
People with HIV can have many complications,
but not everyone does.
If any of these complications happen to you,
doctors will treat them, too.
This is what supportive therapy is all about.

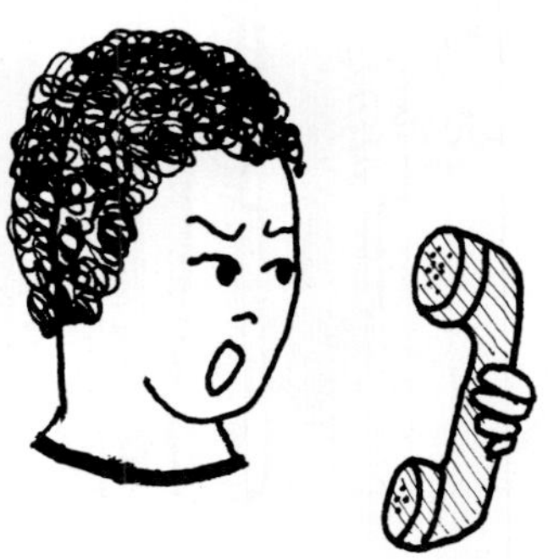

There are ten important complications of HIV infection:

1. Infections

Infections are diseases
that are caused by germs.
Everyone gets them, not just people with HIV.
But, people with HIV get more infections
than other people do,
and these infections can be more serious.
Because people with HIV
have an immunodeficiency,
they also get sick from germs
that don't make most people sick.
The diseases these unusual germs cause
are called "opportunistic infections."
Children are very new people.
They haven't already had lots of diseases
and made antibodies to all sorts of germs.
So, children can have trouble with common infections
that don't bother grownups with HIV much.
This section will tell you a little
about all the different kinds of infections
children with HIV *can* get,
but don't always.

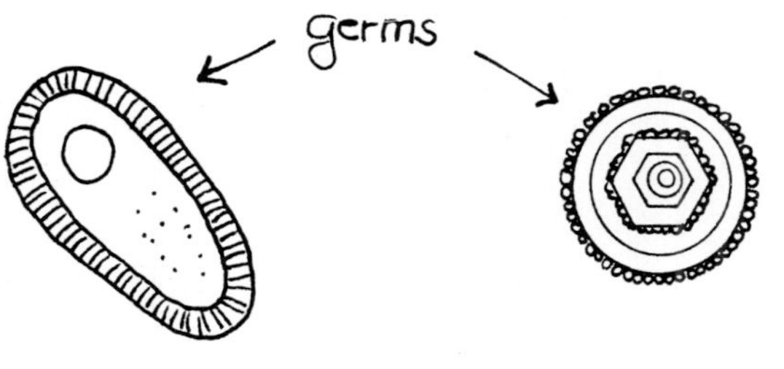

All young children get lots of infections
caused by the kind of germs called "bacteria."
These include otitis media (ear infections),
sinusitis (nose and sinus infections),
tonsillitis, and strep throat.
Children with HIV can get these
as well as other, more serious, bacterial infections
such as regular pneumonia (lung infections),
meningitis (brain infections),
or septicemia (blood infections).
Some bacterial diseases
can be prevented by vaccines (see pages 162-163),
and your doctor will give these to you
if you're old enough.
Another good thing about most bacterial infections
is that they can usually be cured
with medicines called antibiotics.

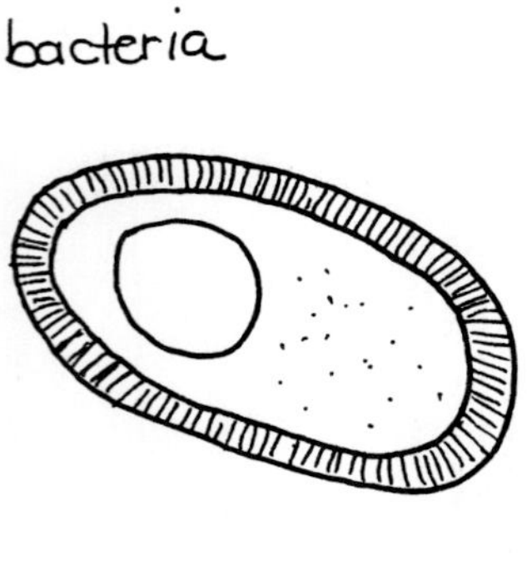

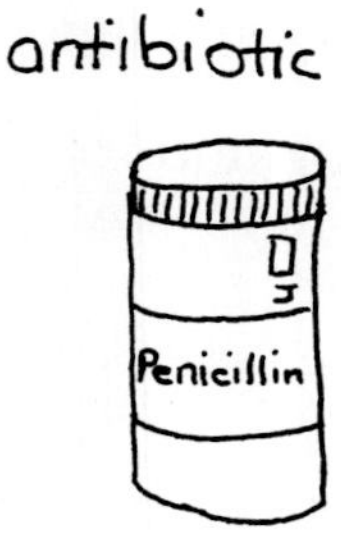

There is one bacteria that has given
people with HIV and their doctors
a lot of trouble.
It is called *"Mycobacterium avium intracellulare,"*
or "*M. avium*" or just "M.A.I.," for short.
It is a cousin of the germ
that causes tuberculosis
(which can also be a problem
for people with HIV).
M. avium can cause you to have
fever, weight loss, tiredness, diarrhea,
tummy aches, big lymph nodes, and just feeling sick.
There are medicines that will kill
the tuberculosis germ
and cure tuberculosis.
But so far, no good medicines have been found
that can kill its cousin, *M. avium.*
If you should get infected by *M. avium,*
your doctors will do all they can
to stop it from bothering you too much,
even though they can't yet cure it.

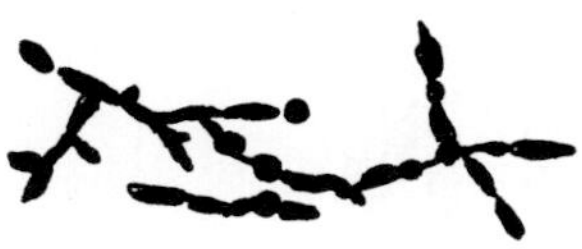
M. avium

All children get lots of infections
caused by the group of germs called viruses.
Viruses cause things like the flu,
measles, polio and chicken pox.
Many diseases caused by viruses

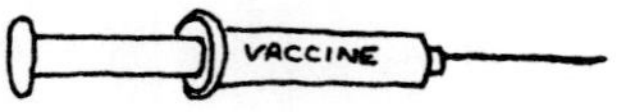

can be prevented by vaccines,
and your doctor will give you these vaccines
if you're old enough
and if the vaccine won't make you sicker.
Other diseases caused by viruses can't be prevented.
Viral infections that many children get
but that can cause special problems
for children with HIV include:
recurrent chicken pox,
chronic EBV (Epstein-Barr Virus) infection,
HSV (Herpes Simplex Virus) infection,
and CMV (Cytomegalovirus) infection.
The kinds of problems these germs cause
depend on the part of the body they infect.
There are antiviral medicines
that can be helpful in some of these diseases.
You can read more about them
at the back of the book.

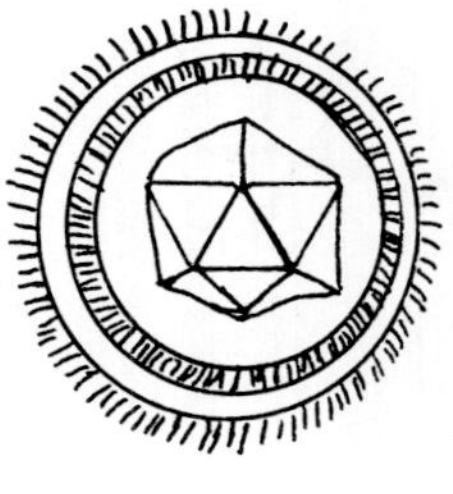

Many children also get infections
caused by the group of germs called funguses.
The most common infection is called "thrush."
It makes your tongue and throat look white,
and it's caused by a fungus called Candida.
It's easy to figure out if you have thrush,
and there are good medicines for it.
These are called "antifungals,"
and you can read more about them
in the back of the book.

Cryptococcus is another fungus
that can cause problems for children with HIV.
This fungus usually infects the brain or the lungs
but it can infect other organs, too.

Other funguses
(or "fungi," if you want to say it right)
that can cause problems for people with HIV
are histoplasmosis and coccidiodomycosis.
These are not very common in children.
Antifungal medicines can be used
to treat all these fungal infections.

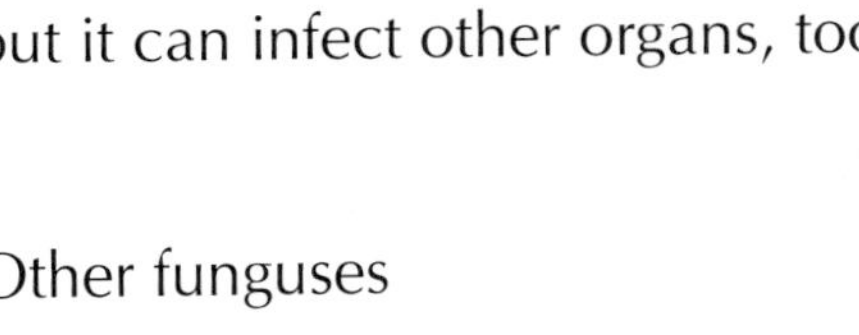

the thrush germ

cryptococcus

Another group of germs
that can infect people with HIV
is the group called parasites.
The parasite that causes the biggest problem
for people with HIV is called *Pneumocystis carinii.*
It causes a kind of pneumonia called PCP,
which is short for "**P***neumocystis* **c***arinii* **p**neumonia."
PCP causes people to have a fever and a dry cough,
and makes it hard to breathe.
PCP can sometimes be cured with antibiotics
or other anti-infective medications
(more about them at the back of the book).
These same medicines are sometimes also used
to help people not get PCP in the first place.
That's a really good idea,
and it can work pretty well.

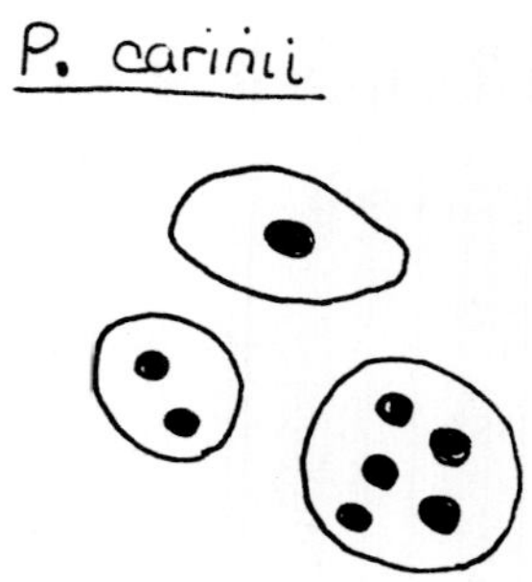

There are other parasites that can cause infections
in children and other people with HIV.
One is *Toxoplasma gondii,* which causes toxoplasmosis.
This is an infection of the brain,
and it can cause fevers, headaches, mixed up thinking,
trouble moving your body when you want to,
or make your body move in ways you don't want it to.
Another is *Cryptosporidium,*
which causes cryptosporidiosis.
Still another is *Isospora belli,*
which causes isosporiasis.
Both of these parasites
infect the digestive system
and cause stomach cramps and diarrhea.
Isosporiasis can be cured with antibiotics.
Cryptosporidiosis is much harder to cure.
Another important kind of treatment for these problems
can be giving your digestive system a rest.
This is done by having you get food and water
intravenously, or IV,
instead of by eating and drinking.
This is often done in a hospital,
but if you have a central line
(see pages 229-235)
you may be able to "eat" this way at home.

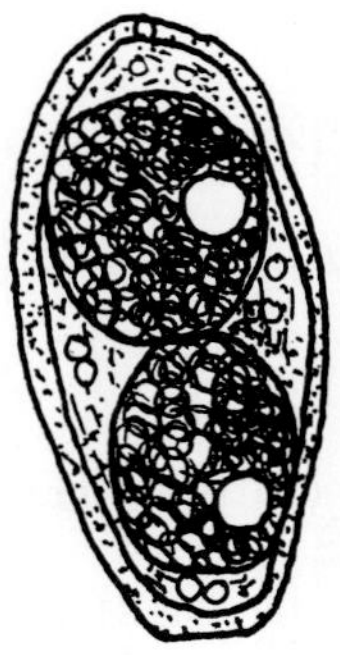

Isospora belli

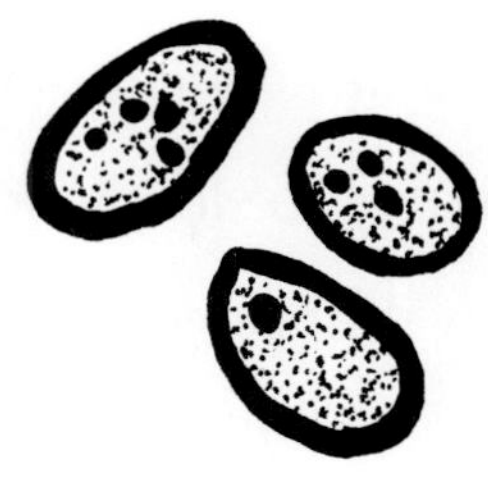

Cryptosporidium

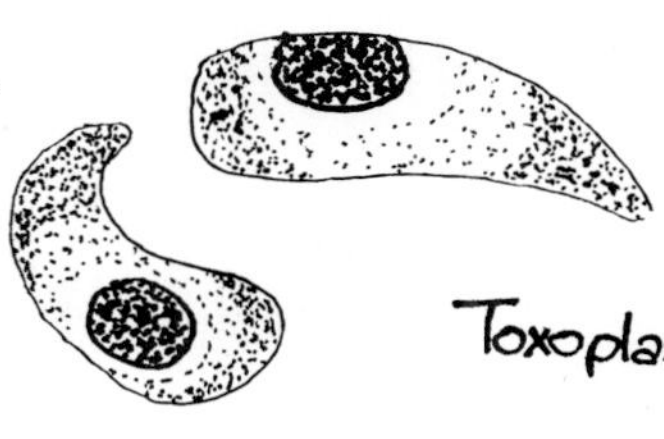

Toxoplasma gondii

There are so many different kinds of infections
that can happen to children who have HIV
that it would take a whole other book
to tell you all about each one of them.
Now you know most of their names,
and that many of them can be treated.
There is one other thing you need to know.
Unlike children who don't have HIV,
you need to call your doctor whenever you get sick.
Maybe it will turn out that all you have
is a dumb old cold.
But, if you have HIV, it could be something else,
and it's probably something treatable.
Any fevers, headaches, stomachaches, earaches,
sore throats, diarrhea, rashes, swollen parts,
throwing up, coughing, bone or muscle or skin aches,
trouble seeing or talking or moving,
being too sleepy or being kind of mixed up—
any of these can mean an infection.
Especially if you were not feeling these things
last week, or yesterday, or even an hour ago.
Don't be afraid to bother your doctor.
Your doctor knows you have HIV
and that if you have an infection,
it needs to be found and treated
right away.

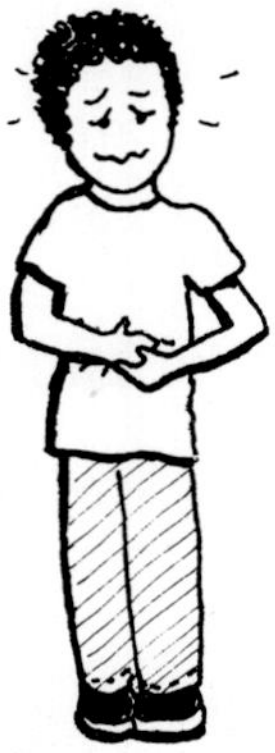

Doctors figure out if you have an infection
lots of different ways.
They can usually find ear infections
just by looking in your ear.
They can see thrush by looking in your mouth.
Other things can't be seen.
Your doctor needs to know
both where your infection is
and what germ is causing it
in order to give you the right treatment.
You can help by telling the doctor
as much as you can about how you feel.
When the doctor examines you,
he or she will get more clues.
X-rays, which are like pictures of your insides,
can also be helpful to the doctor,
and they don't hurt.

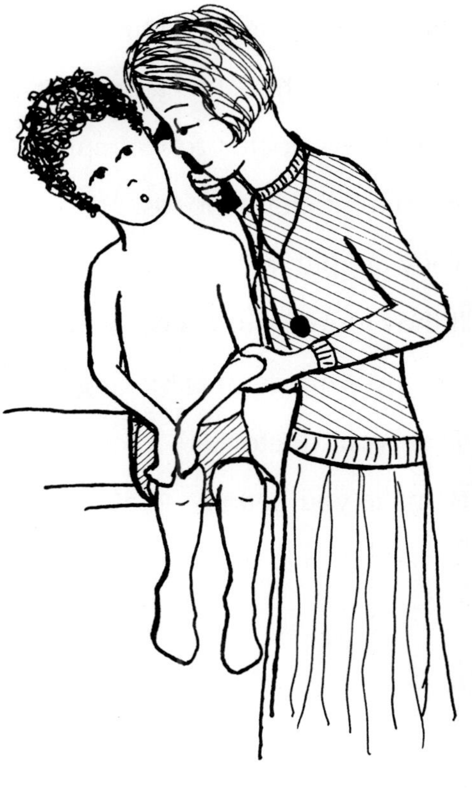

But the best way to know
what germ is causing your infection
is to try to get some of the germs
and grow them outside your body.
This, as you know, is called culturing.
Germs are easier to get from some places
than they are from others.
Getting germs from your skin or throat is easy.
The doctor just rubs something like a Q-tip
on the infected part.
Getting germs from your excretory system
or your digestive system is easy, too.
Your body sends those germs out
in your urine or your bowel movements.
You already know how blood cultures are done,
and that they mean getting a blood test (see page 72).
No matter where the germs come from
or how the doctor gets samples,
the same thing happens.
They are put into a growth medium.
If they grow, your doctor will learn
exactly what germ is making you sick.
Then your doctor will know what medicine you need
to make you better.

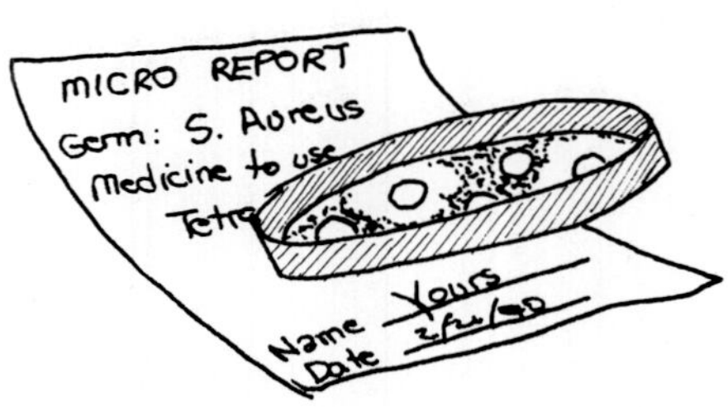

Doctors figure out if you have an infection
lots of different ways.
They can usually find ear infections
just by looking in your ear.
They can see thrush by looking in your mouth.
Other things can't be seen.
Your doctor needs to know
both where your infection is
and what germ is causing it
in order to give you the right treatment.
You can help by telling the doctor
as much as you can about how you feel.
When the doctor examines you,
he or she will get more clues.
X-rays, which are like pictures of your insides,
can also be helpful to the doctor,
and they don't hurt.

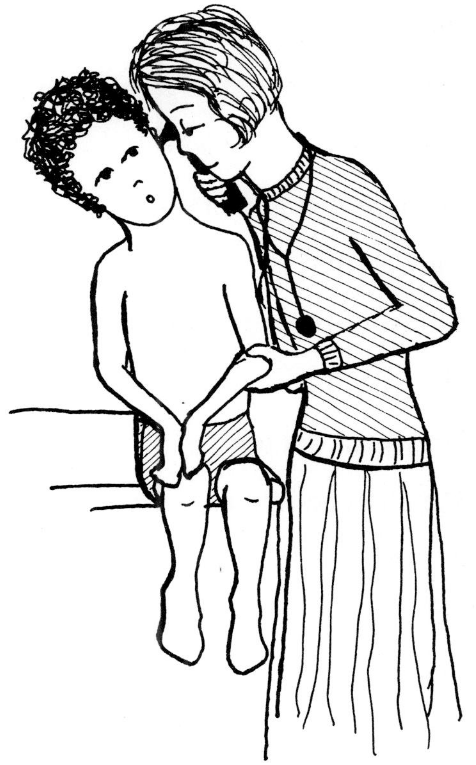

But the best way to know
what germ is causing your infection
is to try to get some of the germs
and grow them outside your body.
This, as you know, is called culturing.
Germs are easier to get from some places
than they are from others.
Getting germs from your skin or throat is easy.
The doctor just rubs something like a Q-tip
on the infected part.
Getting germs from your excretory system
or your digestive system is easy, too.
Your body sends those germs out
in your urine or your bowel movements.
You already know how blood cultures are done,
and that they mean getting a blood test (see page 72).
No matter where the germs come from
or how the doctor gets samples,
the same thing happens.
They are put into a growth medium.
If they grow, your doctor will learn
exactly what germ is making you sick.
Then your doctor will know what medicine you need
to make you better.

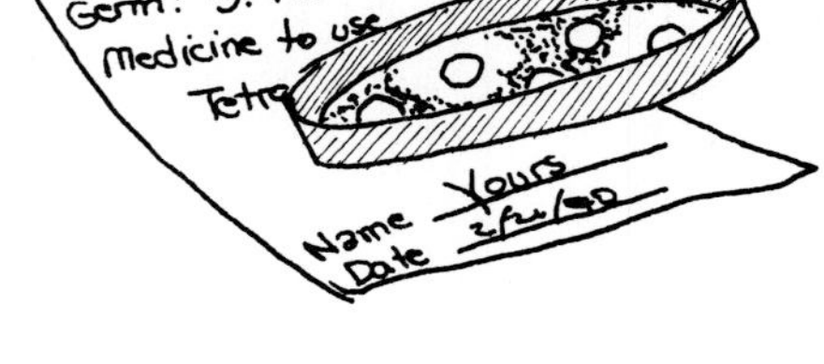
MICRO REPORT
Germ: S. Aureus
Medicine to use
Tetra
Name Yours
Date

You can do a lot to prevent infections.
You can take good care of yourself
by getting enough sleep and food.
Your doctor may be able to give you vaccines
to protect you from some kinds of infections.
You can stay away from people who have infections.
This doesn't mean you shouldn't go to school
or spend time with people you like.
Having fun is another important part
of staying healthy.
It's just that if you know someone has a disease
that you might catch—
or if there's a disease going around your school—
why take chances?
If you are accidentally exposed to a viral disease,
especially chicken pox, regular measles or hepatitis,
be sure to tell your doctor about it.
The doctor may want to give you a shot
that may stop you from getting the disease.

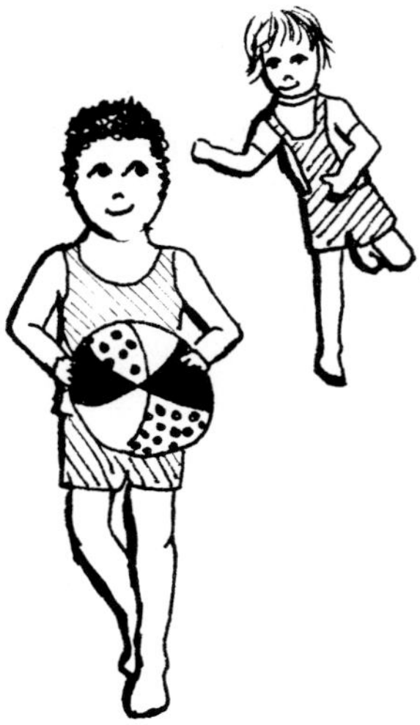

2. LIP

LIP, which is a short way of saying
"lymphoid interstitial pneumonitis,"
is a common problem for children with HIV.
It is a kind of pneumonia, or lung infection,
that causes the lungs to fill up with lymphocytes.
No one knows for sure what germ causes it,
but they think it's EBV.
It's usually not as serious as PCP.
The only way to figure out if a person has LIP
is by doing a lung biopsy.
This procedure is described in the back of the book.
Because no one knows what causes LIP,
there is no specific medicine for it.
A medicine that has been very helpful, though,
is called prednisone.
Prednisone is a very old medicine
that has been used in lots of different diseases.
There is more about it at the back of the book.
Oxygen, which comes in a tank like a scuba diving tank
and is breathed in through little nose tubes,
can also help people with LIP feel better.
So can medicines called bronchodilators,
which can make it easier to breathe.

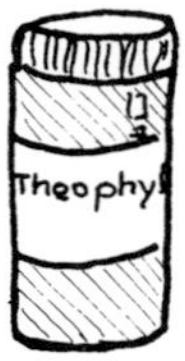

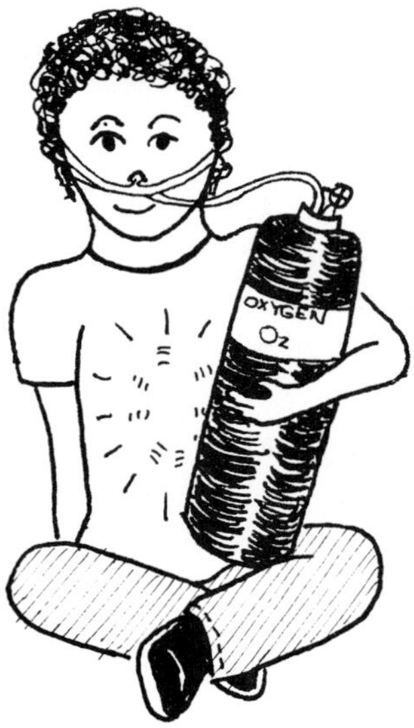

3. Anemia (see pages 21, 74-76)

A lot of people who have HIV get anemia.

Anemia means one of two things:

either you don't have enough red blood cells (RBCs),

or they are not doing a good job carrying oxygen.

People who have anemia

look very pale and feel tired and weak.

Doctors figure out if you have anemia

by doing a blood count.

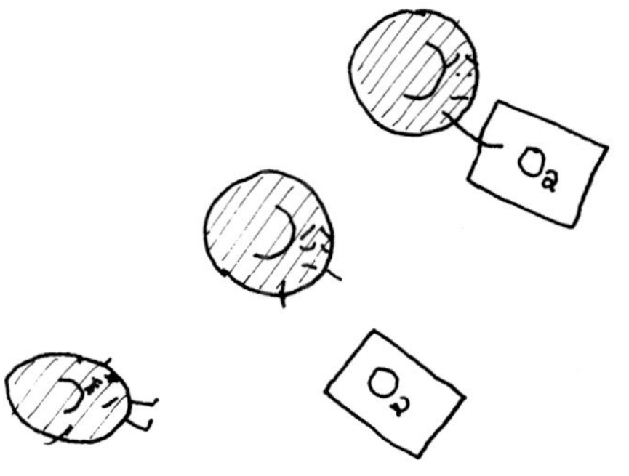

Anemia can be caused by HIV.

It can be caused by other infections.

It can be caused by some medicines.

It can be caused by a poor diet.

Whatever causes your anemia,

your doctors will try to fix it.

They may ask you to eat a special diet

or to take certain vitamins or iron.

They may want to change your medicines for a while.

Or, if your anemia makes you too tired and weak,

they may want you to have a blood transfusion

(see pages 221-228).

A blood transfusion is kind of like

a reverse blood test.

Instead of blood being taken out of you,

blood is put into you,

giving you the RBCs you need to carry oxygen.

4. *Thrombocytopenia* (see pages 22, 74-76)

Thrombocytopenia is when
you don't have enough platelets.
Without enough platelets,
your blood vessels get leaky.
You can bleed inside your skin,
which is what a "black and blue mark," or bruise, is.
You can get nose bleeds
or bloody gums when you brush your teeth.
Or, your tiniest blood vessels can leak,
and you might get little red spots,
like freckles, on your skin.
These are called petechiae.
Or, you could start to bleed inside your head,
which could give you a headache, blurry vision,
or even make you faint.
(If something like this happens, you should call your doctor
and go to the hospital right away.)
As with anemia, if your platelet count gets too low,
your doctor might want you to have
a kind of blood transfusion that is mostly platelets.

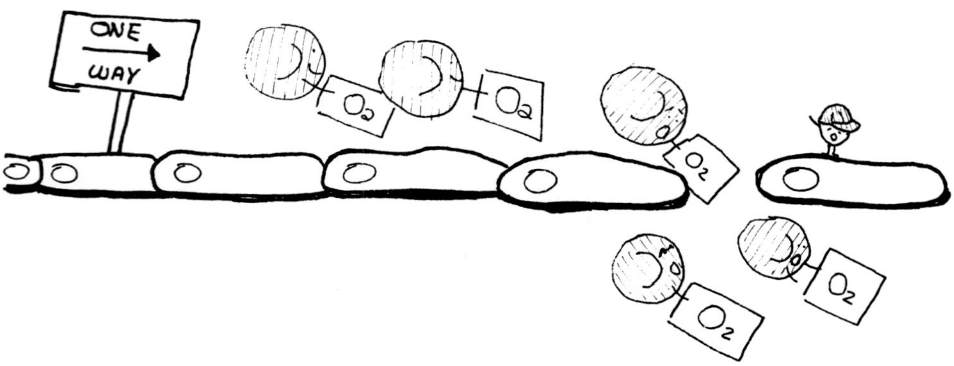

5. CNS Complications (see page 18)

CNS is a short way of saying "central nervous system."

This is your brain and spinal cord.

Your spinal cord is like a strong rope,

and it's made of the big nerves that go to and from the brain.

You already know about a lot of things

that can happen to the CNS in children with HIV.

You know that some germs cause brain infections,

such as toxoplasmosis or CMV.

You know that if you don't have enough platelets,

you can have bleeding in your brain.

But you may not know,

because doctors didn't know it for a long time,

that HIV can infect cells in the brain.

Some brain cells wear the CD-4 antigen.

HIV infection of brain cells can cause headaches

and a lot of the same troubles the other CNS complications do.

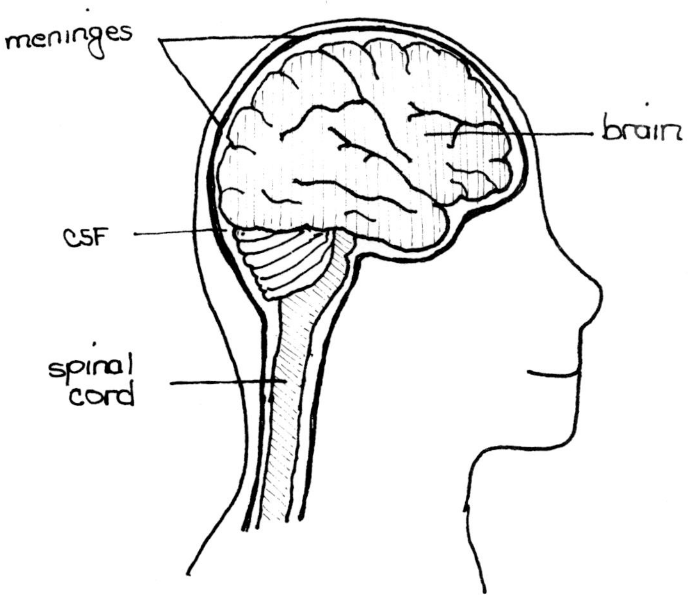

The main trouble it causes is forgetting.
The brain is where we do all our remembering,
but people whose brains are infected with HIV
can do more forgetting than remembering.
They can forget little things,
like what they had for dinner.
Or bigger things,
like the words to their favorite song.
Or really important things,
like how to walk
or how to talk.
These kinds of forgetting
can make people feel angry, sad, or frustrated.
AZT, one of the medicines used to slow down HIV,
has been very helpful with this forgetting problem,
especially in children.
If you are having trouble remembering things,
be sure to talk to your doctor about AZT
if you are not taking it now.

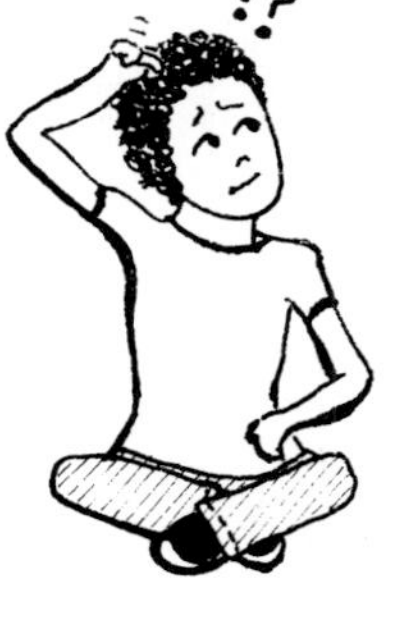

Seizures are another CNS complication
that some people with HIV have.
Seizures are when the brain
makes parts of the body move around for no reason.
Seizures aren't so bad for the person who has one,
although he or she often feels mixed up and sleepy afterwards.
In fact, if you have a seizure,
you won't even know it until someone tells you.
But seizures can be really scary
for the people who watch them.
For this reason,
and because you can get hurt
if you fall down and bump yourself during a seizure,
your doctor will probably want to give you a medicine
so you won't have more seizures.
There are lots of good medicines for this.
The ones used most often for children
are phenytoin (Dilantin) and phenobarbital.

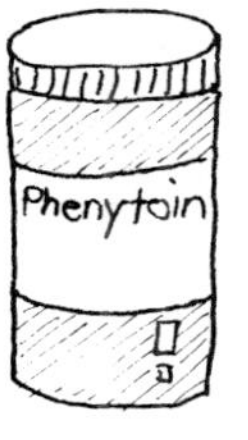

Meantime, if you have a seizure,
your parents or caretakers should know
that they need to do two things.
One is to try keep you from hurting yourself
during the seizure.
The other is to call your doctor.
Most seizures don't last very long,
only a few seconds or minutes,
and you will be OK when it's over.

6. Digestive System Complications (see page 12)

Your digestive system
is like a long tube that goes from
your mouth—where you put food in—
to your anus—where the stuff in food
that your body can't use
comes out when you have a bowel movement.
There are two main problems
people with HIV can have
with their digestive systems.

One is called "anorexia,"
which just means not being hungry enough
to eat enough
to grow and gain weight and stay healthy.
Most people who are sick
don't feel like eating as much as usual,
not just people with HIV.
But all people who are sick
need to eat even when they don't feel like it,
especially children.

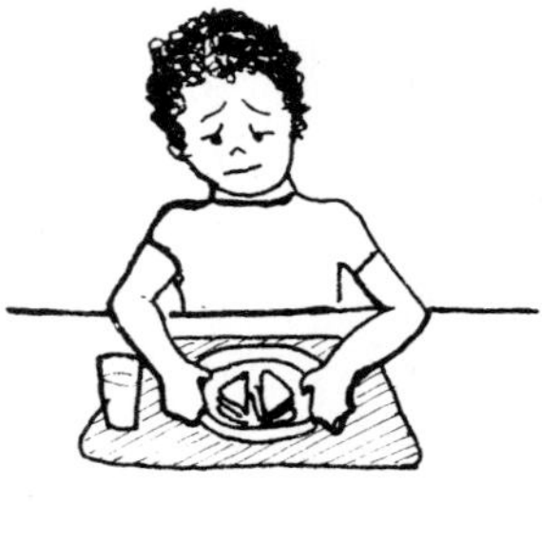

The other digestive system problem
that many people with HIV can have is diarrhea.
Diarrhea is when you have
bowel movements that come too often
or too fast or are too runny.
Besides being a big bother,
diarrhea often means that the food you eat
is going through your body so fast
that your digestive system doesn't have time
to get all the good stuff out of it.
So, even though you're eating,
your body is not getting what it needs.
Diarrhea can be caused by an infection,
by a medication, or by HIV itself.
If you have diarrhea,
your doctors will want to figure out why
and will fix the problem if they can.
In the meantime,
you may be asked to eat or drink special foods
to help your digestive system rest and get better.
Or, your doctor may want you
to be fed intravenously (IV) for a while
so your poor digestive system can really get a rest.
You may also need to wear a diaper until you're better.

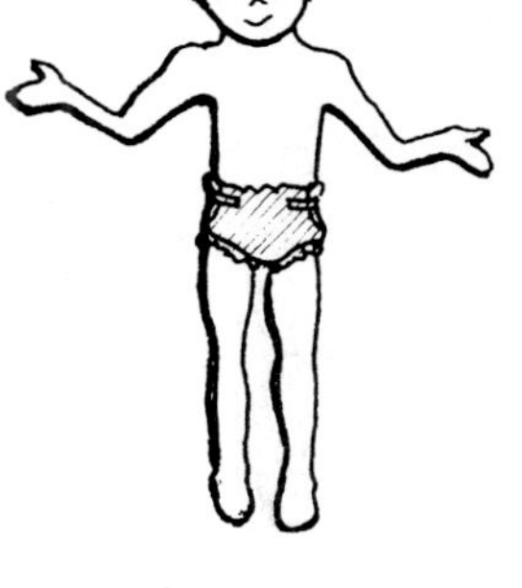

Both anorexia and diarrhea
can cause the people with these problems
to lose weight and not grow right.
You and your parents or caretakers,
as well as your doctors and dietitian,
need to work hard to help you eat well
and help you keep food in your body long enough
for it to be used for growing.
Sometimes you'll get mad at all these grownups
who are trying to make you eat
when you can't or don't want to.
It's OK to have these feelings,
but it's important to let them help you anyway.
As a child, one of your most important jobs
is growing.
All that those bossy grownups are doing
is trying to help you do your job
at a time when it's too hard for you
to do it alone.

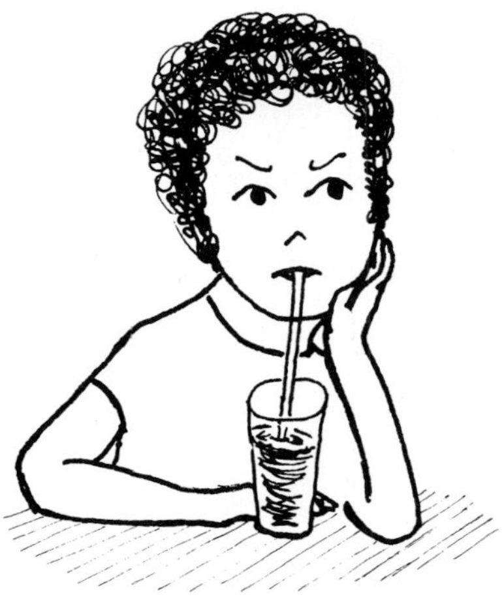

7. Parotitis

If you feel the top of your neck
just under your jaw
you will feel two big soft lumps.
These are called your "parotid glands,"
and they make the watery stuff in your mouth
called saliva.
In a disease called mumps,
which is caused by a virus,
these glands can get so big
that they make the person with mumps
look kind of like a chipmunk.
This can happen to people with HIV, too,
and it seems to happen to children more often
than it happens to adults.
No one knows why this happens,
and there is no real treatment for it.

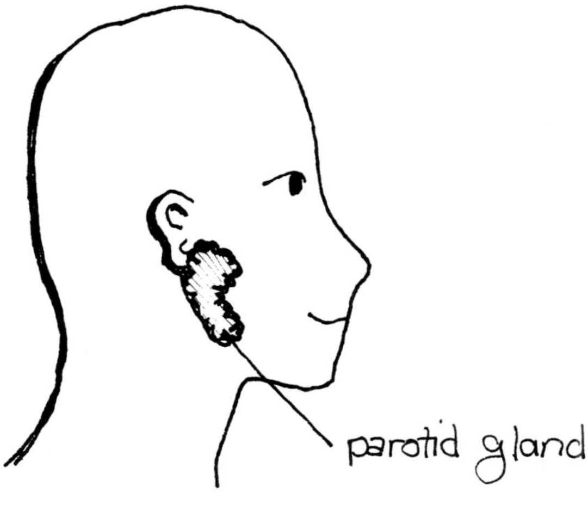

8. Kidney Problems (see page 15)

Your kidneys,

which are part of your excretory system,

can stop working right because of HIV.

No one knows just why this happens.

The symptoms of kidney problems can be:

1. swollen, puffy eyes, fingers, or feet
2. not making enough urine

Often, you will have no symptoms.

Your doctors will only know you have kidney problems

by doing blood and urine tests.

Because no one knows

why people get these kidney problems,

no one has figured out what to do about them yet.

Luckily, this complication isn't very common.

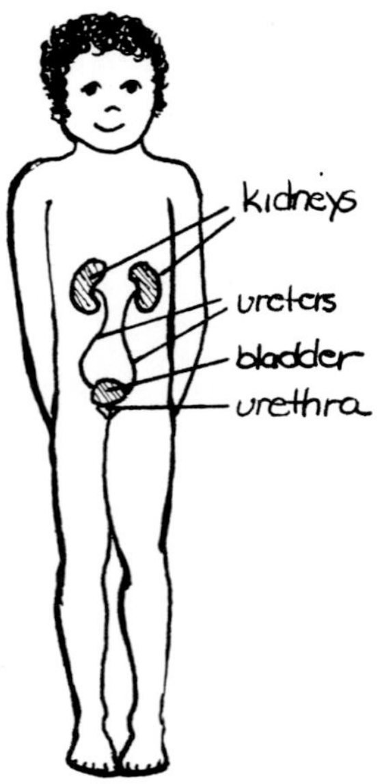

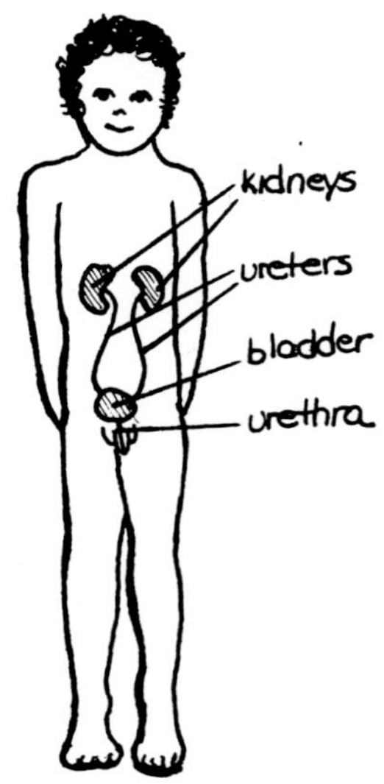

9. Cardiovascular Complications (see page 19)

Some children with HIV

get a kind of heart disease.

The heart is really just a very special muscle.

Sometimes HIV causes the heart muscle

to get tired and weak,

and then it can't do its job of pumping blood

very well.

Symptoms of this complication include:

1. tiredness
2. swollen legs and feet
3. some trouble breathing

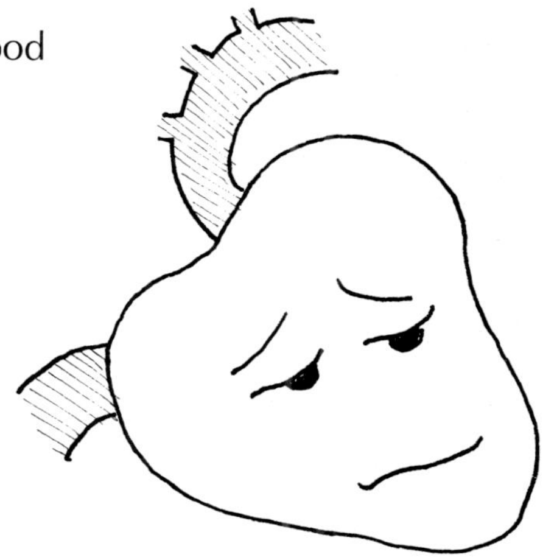

HIV can also affect

the arteries that bring blood to the heart's cells.

This can sometimes cause chest pain.

If you are having any of these problems,

you need to tell your doctor.

Your doctor won't be able

to make the problems go away,

but there are medicines that can help you feel

a whole lot better,

and your doctor may want you to try them.

10. Cancers

Cancers are when a bunch of cells
won't work with the rest of your body.
They get selfish.
They won't follow the rules.
They divide when they feel like it,
which usually isn't when they're supposed to.
They don't do their work right (if they do it at all).
They crowd out normal cells, and the normal cells
can't work right either.
They don't stay in the organ where they belong;
they travel all over the body
and stop and live wherever they like.
They probably don't mean to cause trouble,
but they do.
There are two main kinds of cancer
that happen to people with HIV.
One is Kaposi's sarcoma,
a cancer of the skin and mucous membranes.
This kind of cancer happens often in adults with HIV
but almost never in children.
The other is lymphoma, a cancer of lymphocytes.
This kind of cancer happens often in adults with HIV
and only rarely in children.

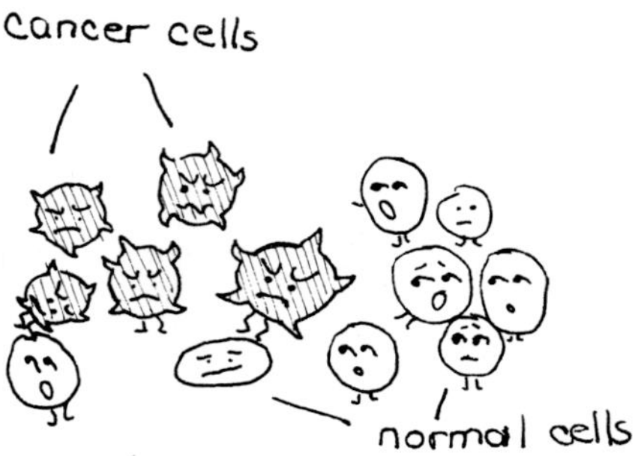

This section on complications
is not meant to worry you.
But it's a good idea
to know about the kinds of problems
that can come up.
You will know—
and your parents or caretakers will know—
when something isn't right with you.
Some people call it "intuition,"
this special kind of knowing.
When you think something is wrong,
please call your doctor.
Some of these complications can be cured,
and most can be treated
so that you will feel better.

And you know something?
Your doctors like to hear about
all the things that go right, too.

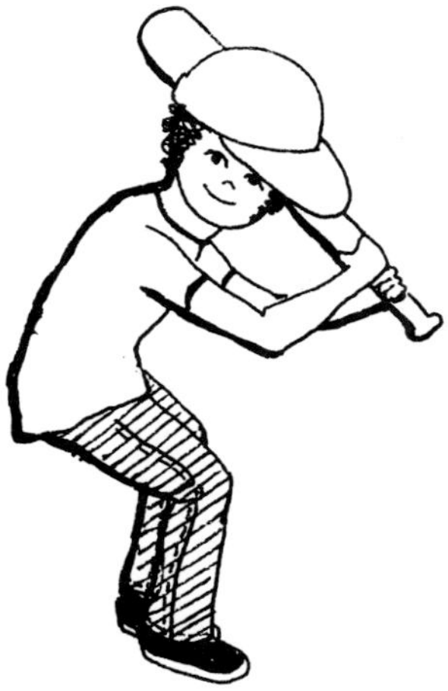

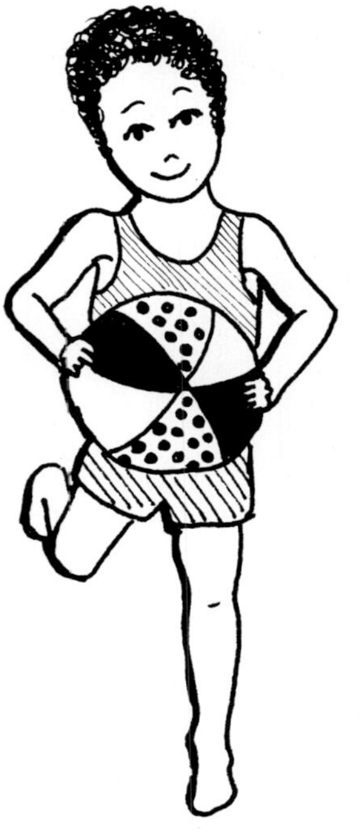

A Day at a Time

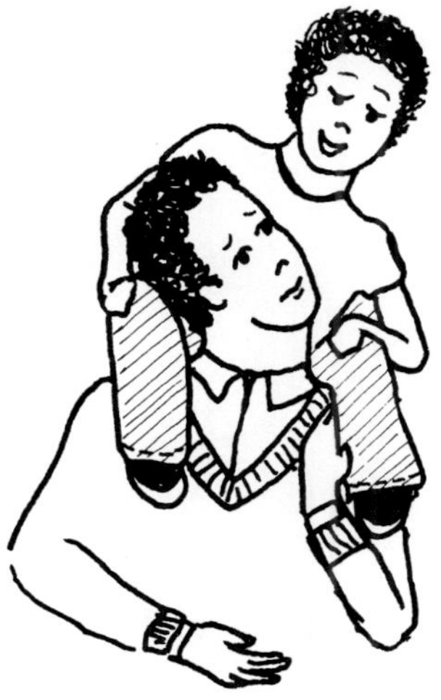

Living with HIV

You will create most of this section for yourself
by living your own life, a day at a time.
Everyone who worked on this book
hopes that your life will be fun and happy.
We hope that you'll feel good most of the time.
We have some suggestions that may help you.
Your life won't be like everyone else's,
but then, no two lives are ever the same.
HIV will change your life.
Not only that, it will affect
the way your family lives.

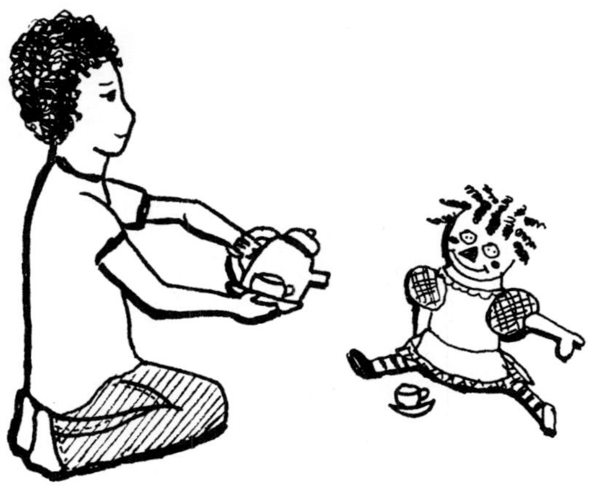

One important way your life will be different

is that you'll go to the doctor and take more medicines

than most people do.

It can be hard to keep track of all this.

One thing that may help

is to use a date book or calendar to keep records.

You can use it to keep track of medicines

that you are supposed to take on certain days and times

and put a sticker to show that you have taken them.

You can keep track of clinic visits, too.

You can also make a list of questions

that you and your parents or caretakers want to ask the doctor.

Or, a list of things you want to tell the doctor.

And, if you take your calendar to the clinic,

you'll be able to mark down any changes in your therapy.

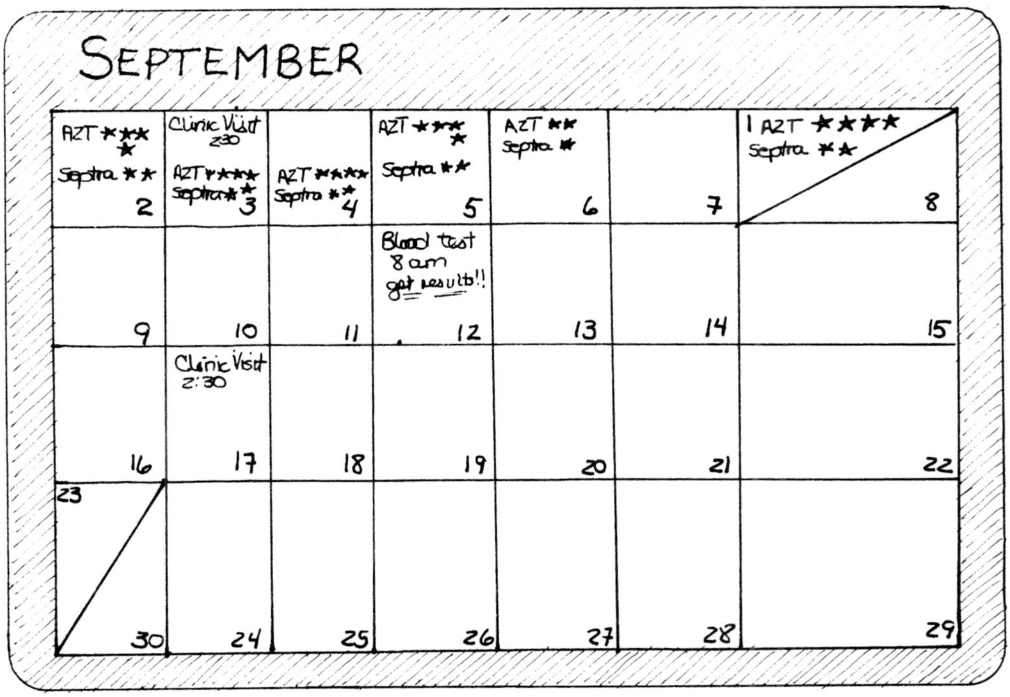

When you go to your clinic visits,
you may want to bring along something to do
like a favorite toy, book or hobby.
Sometimes you have to wait a long time,
and waiting is easier if you have something fun to do.
Or, you might need to have a procedure
that takes a while to do.
Again, the time will pass more quickly
if you bring along some fun things to do.
Another thing you might try
if your parents or caretakers say it's OK
is introducing yourself to other patients and families.
They might not have the same disease as you,
but often they'll be having the same kinds of problems.
You might learn a lot from each other.
You might find someone from your town or neighborhood,
and then maybe you could share rides.
Or you might meet someone
who will become a special friend to you.
You won't know unless you try.
How about it?

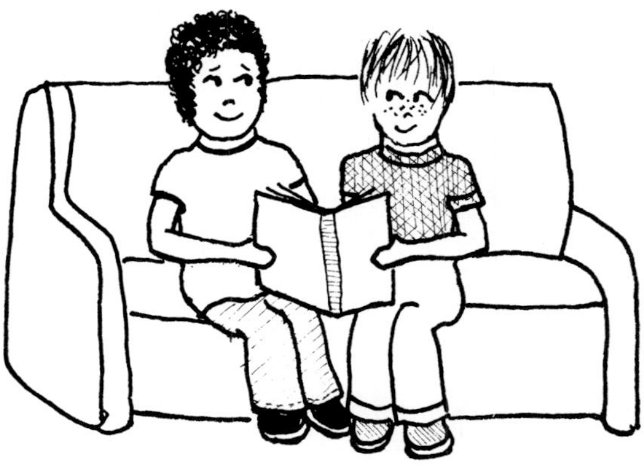

When you go to the clinic or hospital,
you'll see lots of people besides your doctor.
They are all there to help you
each in his or her own way.
You can use the next blank pages
to draw pictures of your clinic friends.
Or, you could ask them for pictures of themselves
and glue them on these pages.
All these different people are interested in you—
not just in your HIV.

The receptionist arranges your appointments
and greets you at every clinic visit.
The receptionist's most important job
is to make sure the doctor has enough time
to spend with you
and all the other patients.

Nurses, like doctors, do many different things.
They may give your medicines to you.
Sometimes they do special procedures, too,
like bone marrow tests or spinal taps.
They have lots of practical advice to give you
about things like what to do about medication side effects.
They are good listeners and good friends,
and often they are specialists
in taking care of people with HIV, like you.

The person who does your blood tests
may be a doctor or a nurse
or a specially trained technician.
If you notice that certain people
are better at doing your blood tests than others,
you might try to schedule your visits
when those people are working.

Special friends that you will have at the clinic
are the social worker, psychologist and psychiatrist.
Some problems just can't be fixed with a shot or pills.
Sometimes you, your parents or your caretakers
need to talk with someone about these problems.
These are the clinic friends who like to talk with people
and who have time just to talk with you.
They can help you get your thoughts together
and be better able to face—and solve—problems.
These friends also know a lot about
the many agencies and organizations
that exist to help people with HIV.
They can teach you how to get the most help
from these other kinds of services.

Another person who will be an important friend
is the dietitian, who is a specialist in food and eating.
Even if you are not having any digestive system problems,
you may want to talk with the dietitian
about how you can eat in the most healthy way
so that you can do your important job of growing.

Medical students, interns, residents and fellows
are all young doctors who are learning about HIV
both from the older doctors—and from you.
In fact, you have a job, too.
Nobody in the clinic is "just" a patient
or "just" a health care professional.
Everyone, including you, is a student
learning about HIV.
And everyone, including you,
has a lot to teach others about HIV.

All of these people together,
plus you and your parents or caretakers,
make up your treatment team.
As with any team, all the members have to work together.
But the goal of your treatment team
is not to win the World Series.
It is to take the best possible care of *you.*

My Treatment Team

My Treatment Team (continued)

Treatment for HIV doesn't just happen
in clinics and hospitals.
It happens at home, too.
In fact, most of your treatment will be done at home,
which is why you and your parents or caretakers
are special members of your treatment team.
One important part of your treatment
is eating enough good food.
Your dietitian can help you learn what to eat,
but it's your job to actually eat it.
That can be hard if you don't feel like eating
or if it hurts to eat.
If you just can't eat anything,
talk to your doctor and dietitian about liquid "foods"
that you can drink instead of chew.
Some of these taste pretty good,
and they can help you get enough vitamins and stuff
until you can eat on your own again.
If you can't even swallow liquids,
talk to your doctor and dietitian about TPN
(total parenteral nutrition).
This is a form of IV feeding that can be done at home
if you have a central line (see pages 229-235).

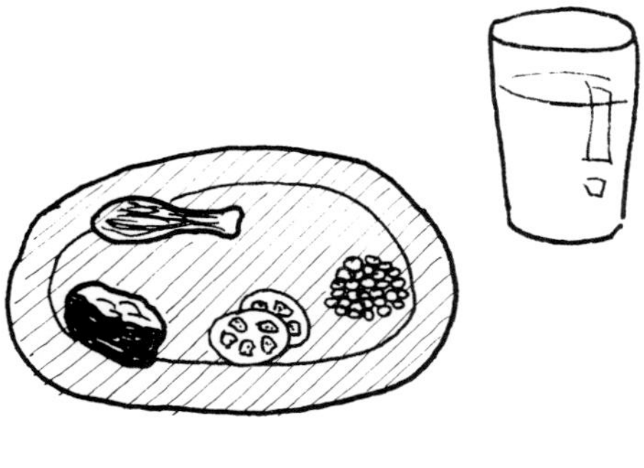

If you get sores in your mouth or throat,
that can also make it hard to eat.
Your doctor may want you to suck on some big pills
(kind of like crumbly cough drops).
These are actually antifungal medicines,
that can make these sores better.
Or, you may be asked to swish a liquid antibiotic
around in your mouth before you swallow it.
Or, your doctor may give you some stuff to swish around
that will make your mouth hurt you less for a while
(but you shouldn't swallow this stuff).
Usually, all these medicines can help you feel better.
But, they don't always taste very good.

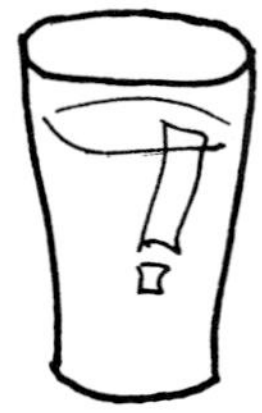

It's also important to get enough to drink,
especially if you are taking TMP-SMX
(also called "Septra" or "Bactrim")
to prevent PCP or to treat some other infection.
It's best to drink a big glass of water or juice
every time you take TMP-SMX.

If you are taking prednisone for LIP,
you should be careful not to eat salty foods.
That will help you not get high blood pressure,
which can be a side effect of prednisone.
Another problem prednisone can cause is heartburn,
which is kind of a hot tummy ache.
If you have this problem, ask your doctor
if you can take an antacid along with your prednisone.

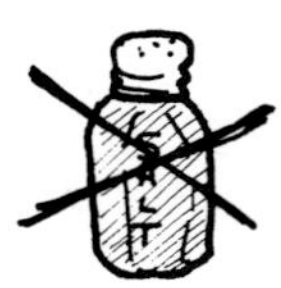

Another thing that can make it hard to eat
is if you are throwing up a lot (vomiting)
or just feeling like you're going to all the time (nausea).
Nausea and vomiting can be caused by many things.
Luckily, there are medications called anti-emetics
that your doctor can give you to help you feel better
even though they can't completely stop the problem.
If you are having trouble with vomiting,
pills can't stay inside you long enough to work,
so the easiest way to take an anti-emetic
is as a suppository.
A suppository is a waxy bullet-shaped pill that,
instead of swallowing (it's too big anyway),
is put just inside your anus (see page 12).
A grownup can give you the suppository
or, if you're older, you can do it yourself.
It's not hard to do and not uncomfortable at all.
And you may feel a lot better.
One important thing about putting in suppositories—
whoever does it should wear latex gloves
which should be thrown away after they're used.
And, of course, hands should be washed
both before and after.

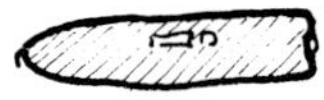

Keeping clean is another important part of home care.
You and your family should just make it a habit
to wash your hands often.
Dishes and food need to be carefully washed, too,
to protect you from infection.
Everyone in the family should have and use
his or her own toothbrush.
If you get a cut, tell a grownup.
The grownup should wash it right away,
and he or she should wear latex gloves.
If any of your blood spilled when you got cut,
it should be cleaned up with
a mixture of water and a little bleach
(ten teaspoons of water and one teaspoon of bleach).
Then the gloves and everything used in the cleanup
should be put in a plastic bag
and be thrown right away.

While most of the things about being clean
are done to protect you from getting infections,
the things about your blood
are to protect others from getting HIV.

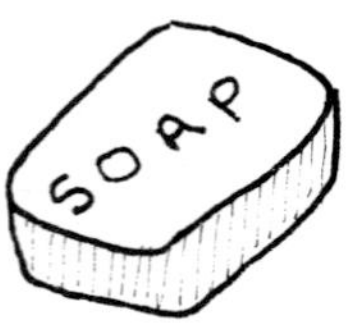

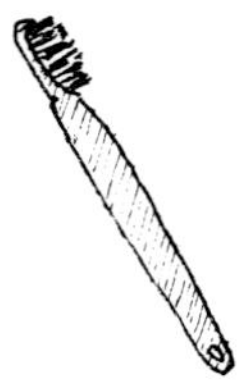

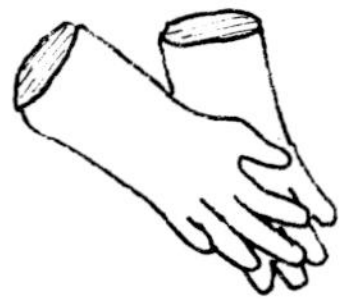

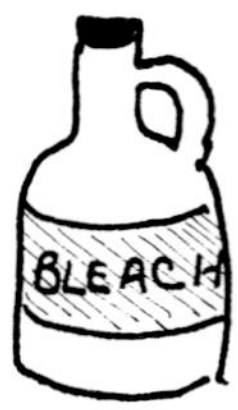

Pain can be another problem for people with HIV.
Sometimes you just have to get through it,
such as the short pain you feel when you have a blood test
or when you bump your head or stub your toe.
Other times, though, the pain can last longer,
and it needs to be controlled.
One way this can be done is by taking medicines
that make the pain hurt less—or not at all.
If you are hurting, you need to tell your doctor.
There are many good medicines for pain.

There are other things that you can do to control pain.
One of them is to use your imagination
to see beautiful things that will help you
relax and forget about the pain.
Another is to use gentle heat,
such as a heating pad (if just a part of you is hurting)
or a warm bath (if your whole body feels badly).
We will say more about pain
in the Special Section on Treatment.
For now, you need to know that pain can be controlled,
and it's something you and your treatment team
need to talk about and plan for.

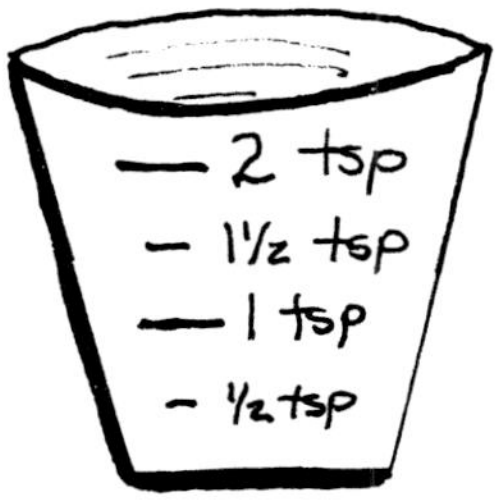

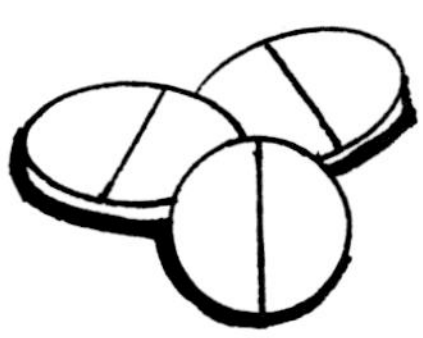

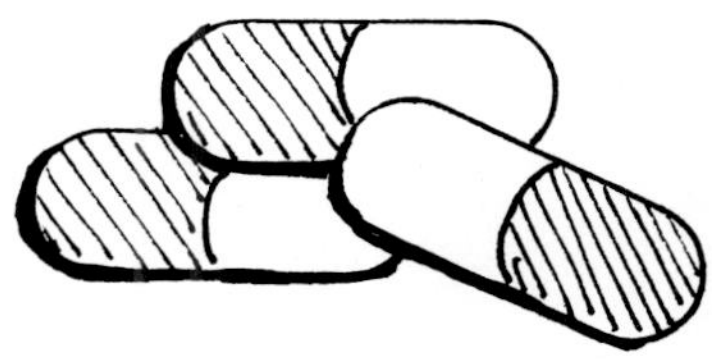

Almost everyone agrees
that the best treatment for any problem
is loving and being loved.
You don't need a prescription for this.
If you're not feeling very good,
try to spend some time with your favorite people
doing quiet things together—
like reading stories or watching T.V.
or playing quiet games.
Your problems won't go away,
but they probably won't bother you as much.

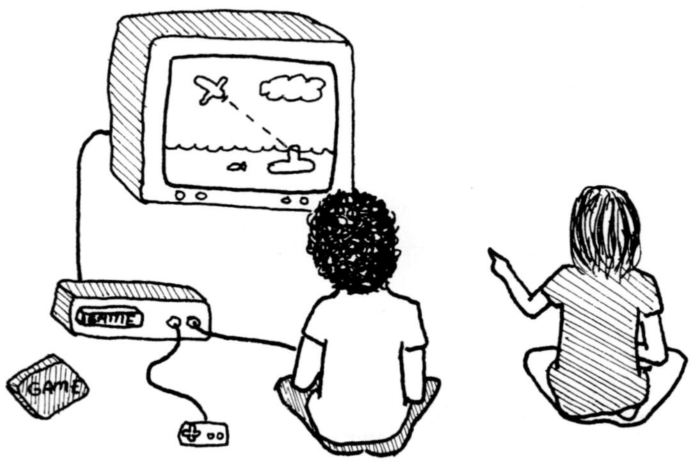

You are part of a family.
We don't know much about your exact family,
but we do know that families get upset
when one or more of them have HIV.
If you have brothers or sisters who do not have HIV,
they may not understand what is happening to you.
They might be afraid that they're going to get HIV, too.
They might think your parents or caretakers
don't like *them* anymore
because they spend so much time with *you.*
You and your parents or caretakers can do a lot
to help your uninfected brothers and sisters
understand your HIV.
You can talk about it with them.
You can invite them to go to the clinic with you
so that they can see what goes on there
and meet all your clinic friends.
You can give them this book to read.
We think that when everyone in a family
understands about HIV and its treatment,
they won't feel left out and scared.
When families are experiencing something
as serious as HIV can be,
it's important that each person within the family
is able to talk about it with the others.

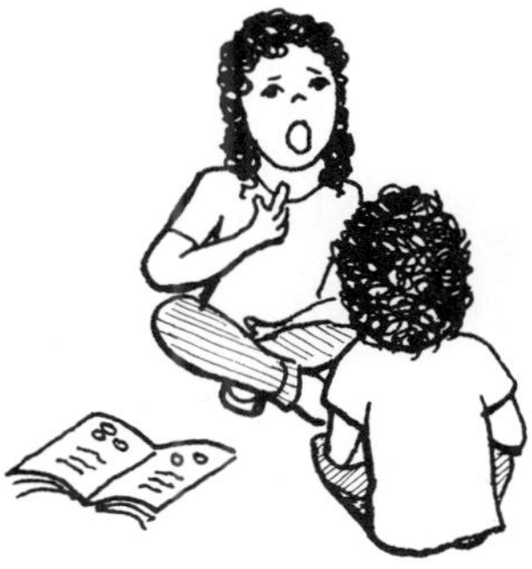

You and your family may have a very big worry.
People with HIV infection don't always live as long as other people.
What if your HIV infection—
or another infection you get because of HIV—
gets out of control?
All of us want to live a long time,
and we want the people we love to have long lives.
So these kinds of thoughts can be very upsetting
to you and to the people who love you.
No one ever thinks anyone they love will get HIV.
When it happens, some people like to pretend it isn't there.
Or, they think they can make it go away
by not talking about it.
You know better than that.
You know that you have HIV
and that it may not always be controllable.
If you pretend it isn't there,
you won't give yourself the very best chance
for a life that is not only long
but full of closeness and happiness.

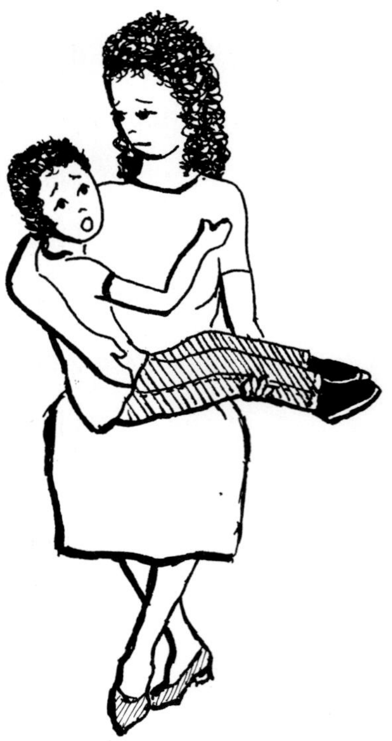

Besides feeling worried,
you and other people in your family
may have other troubling feelings.
For example, you or they may feel angry at times.
The anger might be at your doctors
and the other members of your treatment team
for doing things that you don't like.
The anger may be at God or fate
for making you have HIV when other people don't.
The anger may be at the person
who accidentally gave you HIV.
This can be especially hard for you
if that person was your mother and father.
It's hard because they also gave you your life,
which was a wonderful gift.

Another troubling feeling may be sadness
about not being like other kids
or about maybe not living a long life.
Or a feeling of badness
that there must be something bad about you
for you to have gotten HIV
(even though you *know* better,
these kinds of feelings can still happen).

All these different feelings are normal.
There is nothing wrong with you because you have them,
and it's OK to talk about these feelings
with someone you love and trust.

When you or a member of your family
find that worrying or feelings like anger
are using up a lot of time and energy,
it may help a lot to talk to one another about the worry.
It may help to talk to your doctor or social worker.
If you belong to a religious group,
it may help you to talk to your religious leader.
Sharing your problems and worries
with people you love and trust
is another way of sharing yourself.
It doesn't mean that you are too weak
to take care of your own troubles.
It means that you love others so much
that you want to include them in all parts of your life.
You can help each other not get so worried or angry or sad
that no one has any fun anymore.
It's OK to have feelings about being sick or about dying.
Everyone does.
But try not to be afraid of living
and sharing your life with people you love.
A day at a time.

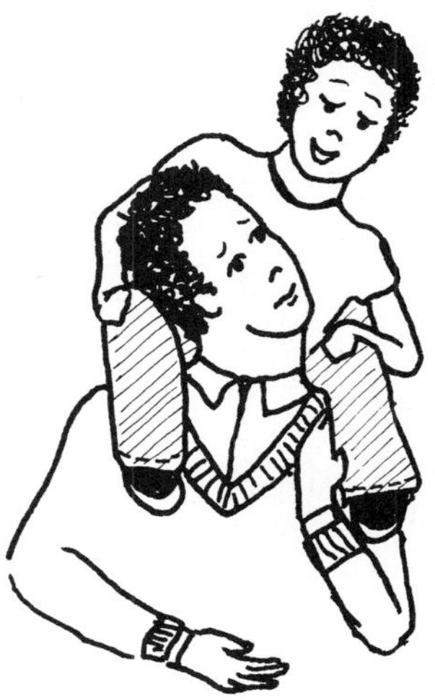

You are also part of a community,
whether it be your block or neighborhood or town or city.
In that community is your school,
your place of worship,
your playground,
your friends,
and other people you see but don't really know.
Some communities have responded in a helping way
to people with HIV,
because they understand the disease
and are not afraid of the people who have it.
Other communities have acted in a hurting way
toward people with HIV,
because they don't understand this disease
and they are afraid of the people who have it.
Your parents or caretakers will probably know
which kind of community you live in.
You need to decide with your family
whom you and they can talk about your HIV with
outside your family.

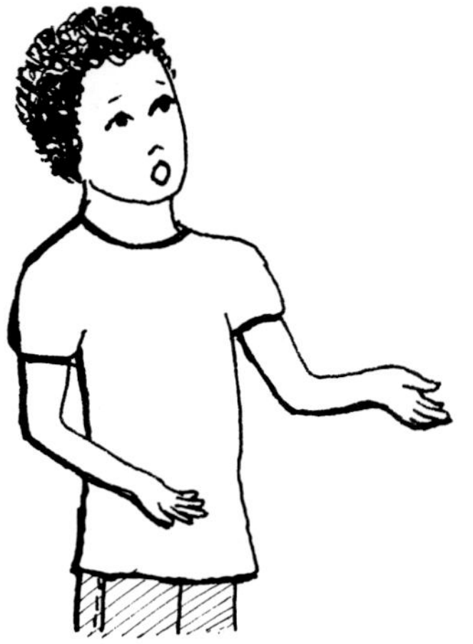

One thing both you and your family should know
is that having HIV
doesn't mean you can't do everything other kids do
as long as you're feeling well enough
and as long as it's all right
with your parents or caretakers.
You can go to school and church and parties.
You can play games and sports.
You can have friends.
You can sing and dance and giggle.
And, just like any other kid,
there are some things you shouldn't do.
You shouldn't get into fights.
You shouldn't bite anyone.
You shouldn't eat food other people have eaten.
You shouldn't share toothbrushes.
Also, just like any other kid,
you don't have to be perfect.
You just have to be the very best possible *you*
that you can be.

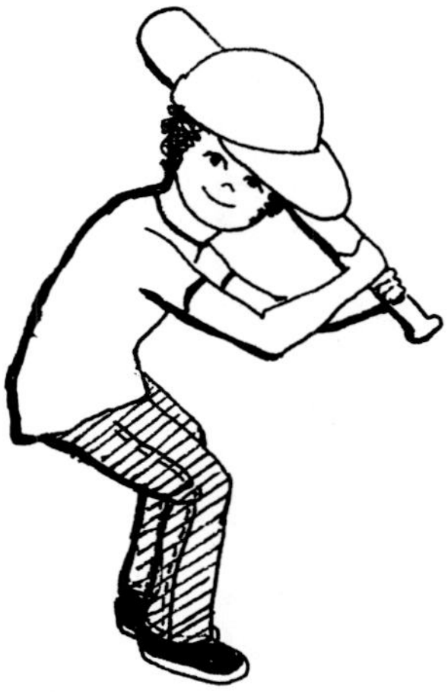

We can't write the rest of this chapter for you.

Only you can do that by living your life

a day at a time.

Other chapters aren't finished either.

"How Doctors Treat HIV" isn't complete yet.

"How To Cure HIV" has only just been started.

A lot of people are working

to find a cure or better treatments for HIV.

At the beginning of this book,

we said you are very special.

You are loved

by both the family you live with

and the larger family of people

who are working to help you live long and well with HIV.

And, just like you,

this group of helping people

is growing bigger all the time.

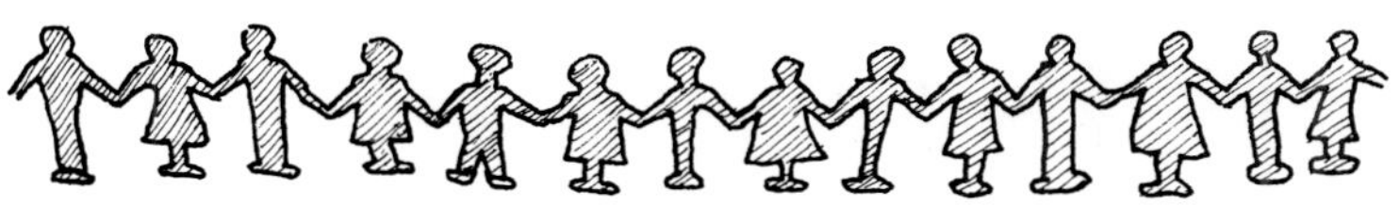

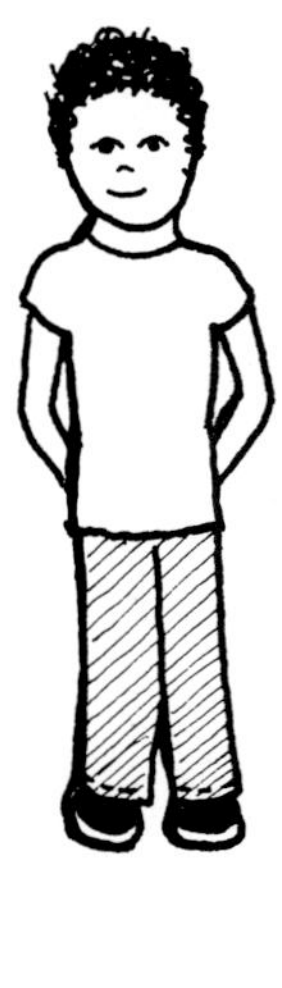

We can't know what the future will hold
either for you or for your HIV.
There are a lot of empty pages in this book
that you can use for your own records.
That way it can keep up with progress
and with you.
If your treatment changes,
you can use the empty pages
to write down your new program.
In fact, you can add whatever you want to.
One warning, though.
If a cure for your HIV is found,
there won't possibly be enough room in this book
for all the pages of your life.
You'll have to start a new book for yourself.
And you know what?
We really hope you have *this* problem!

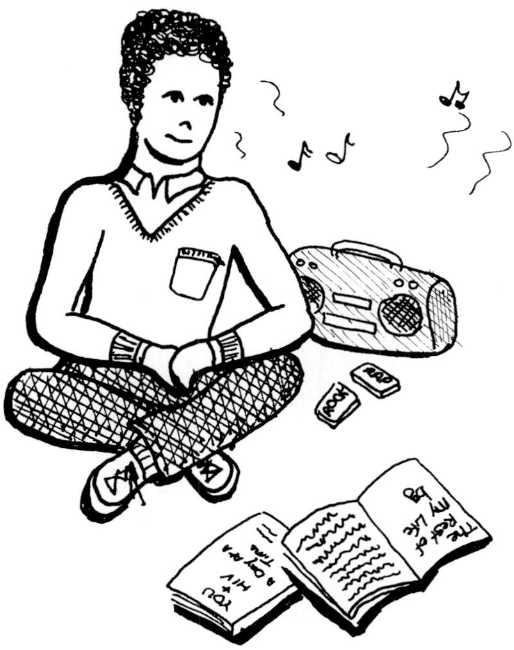

Treatment

things you wanted to know

but didn't think you'd understand

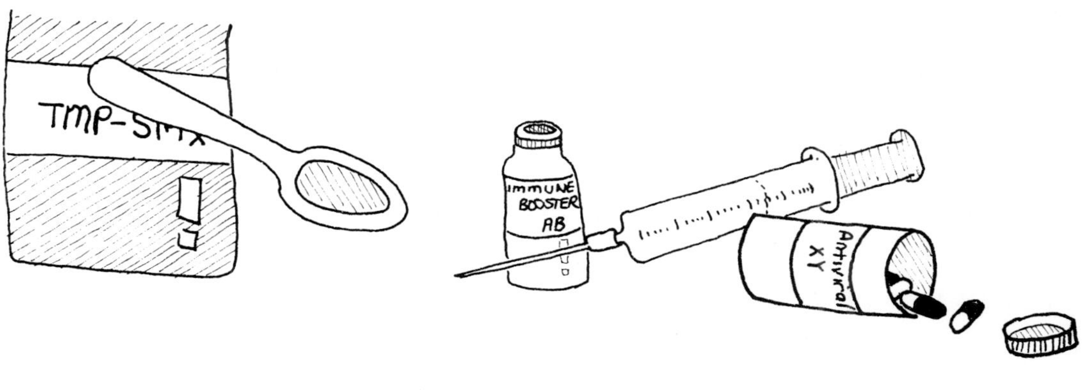

This section of the book

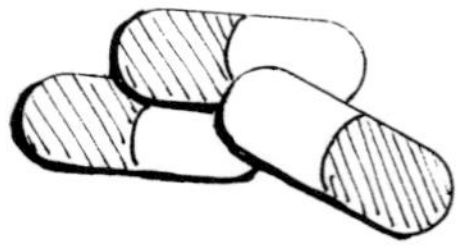

has more details about treatment.

The writer of the book couldn't know exactly

what *your* treatment program would be like.

So, she decided to tell you about

most of the kinds of treatment

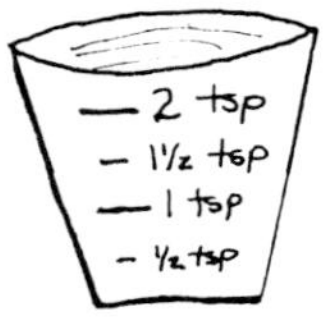

that are now being used or tested.

You can read just the pages

that tell about things that

either have happened or are about to happen to you—

or you can read it all, if you want to.

As you read, it is important to remember

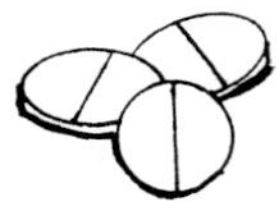

that most of the medicines are still being *tested*

for use in HIV-infected people.

Only a few of them have been *approved.*

All are included in the book

because you may hear about them,

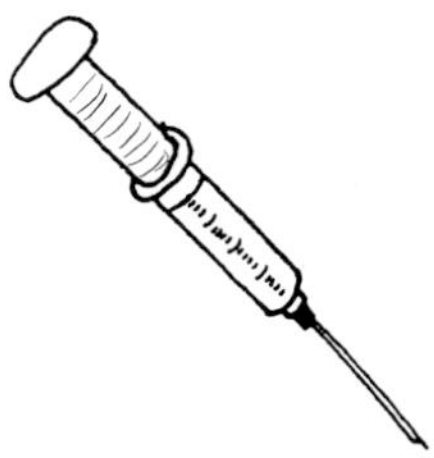

but not because they are known to work.

We are in the early stages of treating HIV,

and most treatments are *very* experimental.

This section can help prepare you

for things that *might* happen.

Just as in the earlier chapter about treatment,

this section will have three parts:

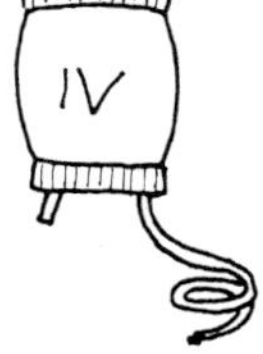

one on antiviral therapy,

one on immune boosters,

and one on supportive therapy.

Antiviral Therapy

Antiviral therapy is medicines that make it hard
for viruses to turn cells into virus factories.
Most of the antivirals you will read about here
are designed to make this hard for HIV.
A few are designed to make this hard
for other viruses you might become infected with.
All medicines, whether or not they are antivirals,
can do other things besides what we want them to do.
These "other things" are called side effects.
Some side effects are unpleasant.
A few are serious.
You may have some side effects—or you may not have any.
It's hard to know.
But if you know about side effects, and you have one,
you don't have to worry.
You'll know it's not your HIV getting worse.
You and your doctors will watch for these side effects.
Some of them can be found by doing blood tests
or bone marrow tests (see pages 172-176).
Others can be seen when the doctor examines you.
Others you will just have to tell the doctor about.
If you have serious side effects,
your doctor may want you to take less
of the medicine that is causing them—or none at all,
for a while.

Besides side effects,

each of the medicines you take

can affect how the other ones work.

Sometimes they help each other work better.

Sometimes they make it harder for each other to work.

Sometimes they make another medicine's side effects worse.

Because of this, you need to tell

every single doctor or dentist that you see

about every medicine you are taking

so they don't accidentally give you a new medicine

that will cause problems with the old ones.

And, because of this, you should never take any medicine—

even something you buy off the shelf at a drugstore—

without talking to your doctor about it first.

All medicines are powerful,

not just the ones you need a prescription for.

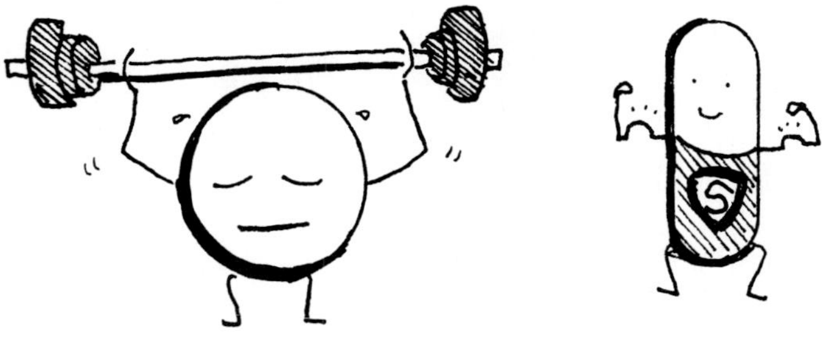

AZT

is also called zidovudine, ZDV,
azidothymidine or Retrovir.
It can be given as a pill or a syrup
or intravenously (IV).
It has been *approved* to treat HIV in adults and children.
It works by slowing down reverse transcriptase,
the put-together enzyme HIV uses to make proviral DNA.
It is given every day, usually every six hours.

Side effects that AZT can cause are:

1. low granulocyte counts (see pages 24, 75)
2. anemia (see page 109)
3. headaches
4. nausea
5. trouble sleeping
6. muscle aches

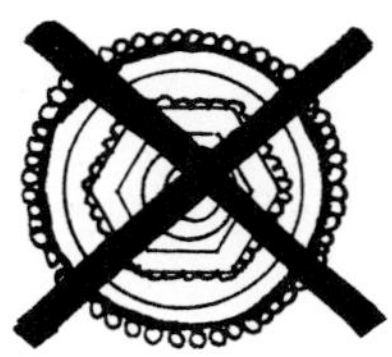

Other medicines that may not get along with AZT are:
dapsone, pentamidine, trimethoprim-sulfamethoxazole,
amphotericin B, flucytosine, interferon,
acetaminophen, aspirin, indomethacin and phenytoin.
Most of these medicines are talked about in this book.
Because you may need to take one or more of these medicines
along with your AZT,
you and your doctor will have to watch you closely
to be sure they get along.
Two medicines that may help AZT work better
are quinine and probenecid.

ddI

is also called dideoxyinosine.

It can be given as a liquid or IV.

It is being *tested* to treat HIV in adults and children.

It works by slowing down reverse transcriptase,

the put-together enzyme HIV uses to make proviral DNA.

It is taken every day,

once, twice, or three times a day.

Side effects that ddI can cause are:

1. pancreatitis, which starts as a stomachache
   with nausea and vomiting
2. mild headache, when given IV
3. rash
4. tingly, burning, or achy legs and feet

Most children don't have trouble with side effects from ddI.

ddI is so new that no one knows for sure

how other medicines will react with it.

Two medicines that it may not get along with

are trimethoprim-sulfamethoxazole (TMP-SMX)

and ketoconazole.

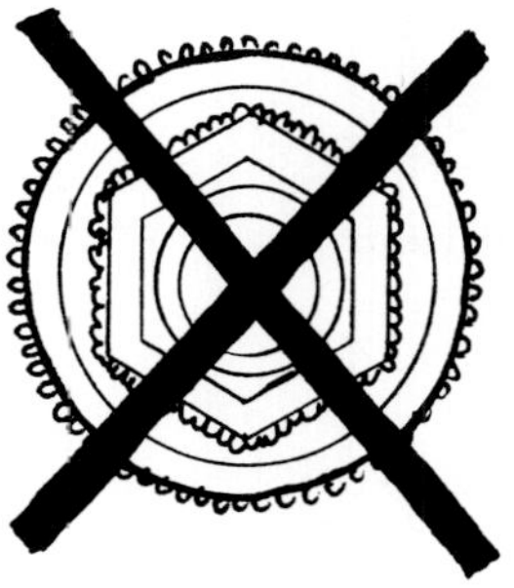

There are a number of other medicines
that also work by slowing down reverse transcriptase,
just as AZT and ddI do.
At this time, only one of these medicines
is being *tested* in children.
It is called ddC (dideoxycytidine),
which comes as a pill or IV.
ddC can make some people feel kind of sick
when they first take it,
but this sick feeling goes away.
Another side effect that has happened to adults
is tingly, burning, or achy legs and feet.

There are two other medicines that work like ddI and ddC
that are now being *tested* in adults.
We thought you might like to know their names
even though they haven't been found safe or useful enough yet
to be tried in children.
They are: AzdU (Azidouridine, AzUrd)
which comes as a pill or IV;
and d4T (2'3'-dideoxythymidinene)
which comes as a pill or IV.
Side effects of these medicines are not yet well known.
Nor is much yet known about how these medicines act
when mixed with other medicines.

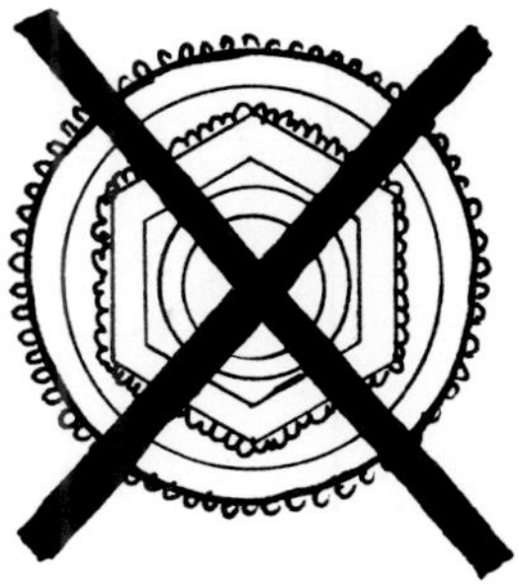

Soluble CD4

is also called CD4 or rCD4.

It is given IV

or as a shot into a muscle (intramuscular or IM)

or as a shot just under the skin (SC or Sub-Q).

It is being *tested* to treat HIV in adults and children.

It is given on an irregular schedule,

sometimes every day, sometimes not.

It works by stopping HIV from infecting cells.

CD4 has not yet been shown to have

any serious side effects in people.

Other medicines that work like CD4

that are now being *tested* in adults are:

CD4-IgG, which is CD4 attached to an antibody

and can not only block HIV from infecting cells

but also kill cells that are already infected;

and Peptide T, which attaches to the CD-4 antigen

on uninfected cells

blocking HIV from infecting them.

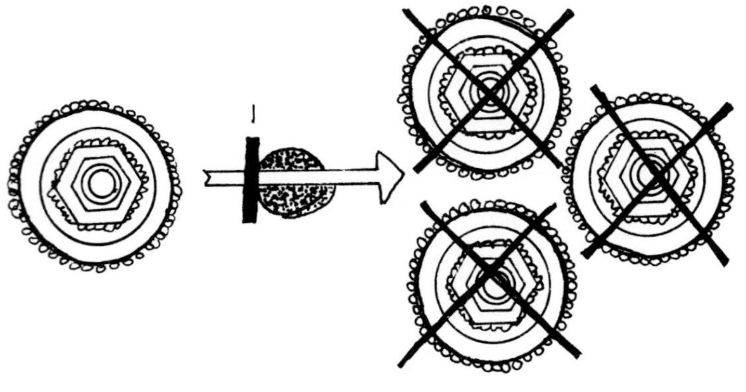

A number of other medicines are or have been
tested in adults with HIV.
Because you may hear about them,
they will be listed here.
But it is important to remember
that they are not even being tested in children now,
because they either haven't worked in adults
or they haven't been found to be safe yet.
These are: ribavirin,
which has many other names;
butyldeoxynojirimycin,
which is also called N-Butyl-DNJ or NbuDNJ;
diethyldithiocarbamate,
which is also called DTC;
AL-721; dextran sulfate;
GLQ.223,

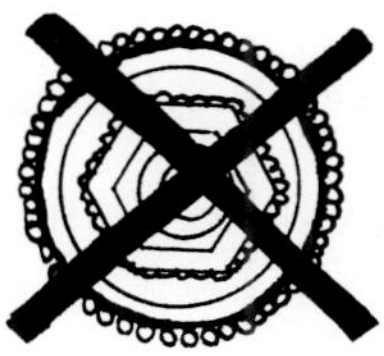

which is also called Compound Q
(because it comes from a kind of cucumber);
and HPA-23.

Again, *these medicines have not been tested in children*
and many have not been found to be helpful for adults.
Even so, this list tells you something important—
that scientists and patient volunteers are working hard
to find medicines that will be safe
and that will work
for you.
It's just that not everything they try works out.

Acyclovir

is also called Zovirax.

It comes as a pill, an ointment or IV.

It is *approved* to treat herpes infections in everyone

and is being *tested* to treat chicken pox

and other viral infections in people with HIV.

It is also being *tested* in combination with AZT

to treat HIV infection itself in adults.

It works by stopping the herpes viruses

from making more of themselves,

and probably does the same thing

with the chicken pox virus.

It is given IV three times a day

to children with HIV who have chicken pox.

It can also be given as a pill up to five times a day

to prevent the chicken pox from coming back.

Side effects that acyclovir can cause are:

1. kidney problems
2. pain and swelling at the place the IV went in
3. nausea and vomiting
4. rash
5. sweating

Other medicines that may not get along with acyclovir are:

AZT and probenecid.

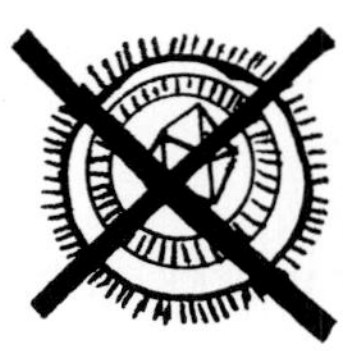

Vidarabine

has many other names.

It is given IV.

It is sometimes used to treat herpes infections

when acyclovir doesn't work.

It works by stopping the herpes viruses

from making more of their DNA plans.

Vidarabine causes lots of side effects in adults,

but it doesn't bother little children as much.

Side effects vidarabine can cause are:

1. loss of appetite
2. nausea and vomiting
3. diarrhea
4. headache
5. mixed up feeling
6. dizziness
7. shakiness
8. rash

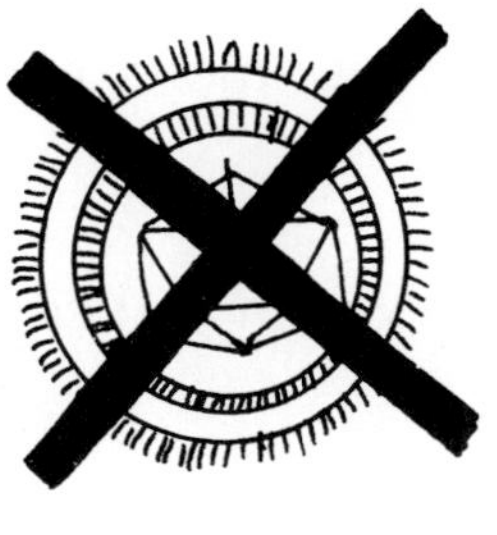

Ganciclovir

is also called Cytovene or DHPG.

It is given IV.

It is *approved* to treat eye infections caused by CMV

and is being *tested* to treat

infections caused by close relatives of CMV, such as EBV.

It works by stopping the CMV

from making more of itself.

It is given twice a day for several weeks.

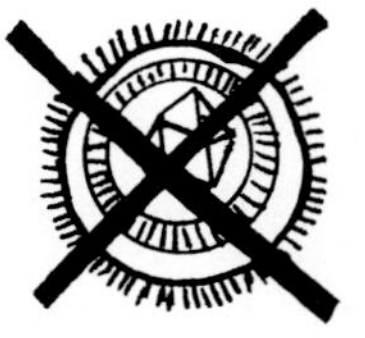

Side effects that ganciclovir can cause are:

1. low granulocyte counts
2. low platelet counts (see page 75)
3. anemia
4. liver problems
5. kidney problems
6. confusion

Other medicines that may not get along with ganciclovir are:

AZT, dapsone, pentamidine, amphotericin B,

trimethoprim-sulfamethoxazole, and probenecid.

Because you may need to take one or more of these medicines

along with your ganciclovir,

you and your doctor will have to watch you closely

for side effects,

and one or more of the other medicines

may have to be stopped for a while.

Foscarnet sodium

is also called just Foscarnet.

It is given IV.

It is being *tested* to treat CMV and other viral infections

in people with HIV.

It is also being *tested* in combination with AZT

to treat HIV infection itself in adults.

Side effects that Foscarnet can cause are:

1. kidney problems
2. low hemoglobin count (see page 75)
3. tiredness and crankiness
4. shaking
5. headache
6. pain and swelling where the IV was put in

Other medicines that may not get along with Foscarnet are:

certain antibiotics, pentamidine, and amphotericin B.

A medicine that can work better with Foscarnet

is AZT.

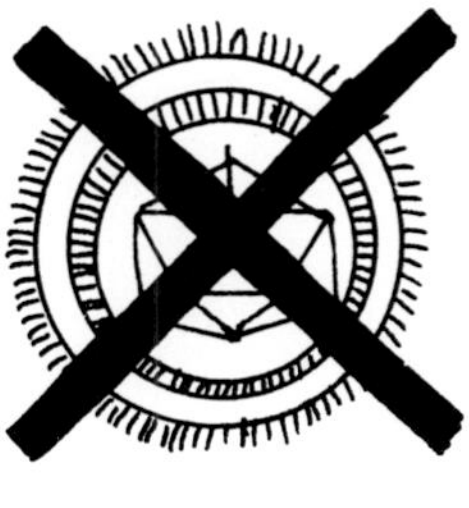

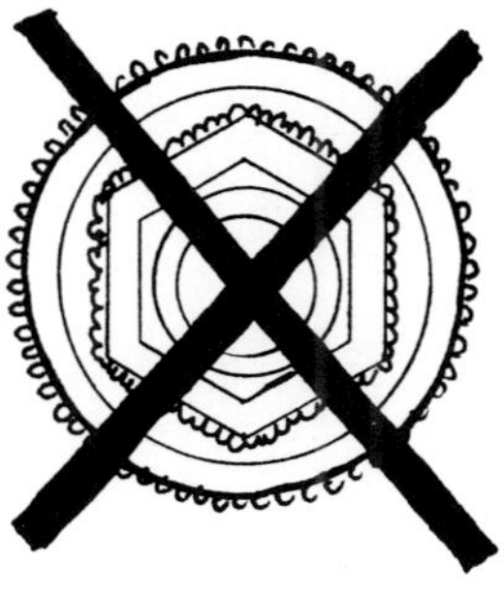

There are other antivirals you may hear about
that have not been discussed here.
That is because at the time this book was written,
these were not being tested in the United States,
or because they haven't been discovered yet.

The rest of this page and the next
are for you to use
to write down information about any new antiviral medicine
you might hear about or take.

New Antiviral Medicines

New Antiviral Medicines

Immune Boosters

You have learned a lot about your immune system.
You have learned that its goal
is to protect your body from germs.
You have learned that it's made up of
many different kinds of cells
and that these cells all have different jobs to do
in your body's defense.
You have learned how your immune system
can figure out which cells are yours and which are not,
depending on their antigens,
and what the different parts of the immune system do
when they run into a cell with the wrong antigens.
Given all that you have learned
about what the immune system does,
you can probably guess
what immune boosters are.
Immune boosters are treatments
designed to help your immune system
do a better job in fighting your HIV infection.

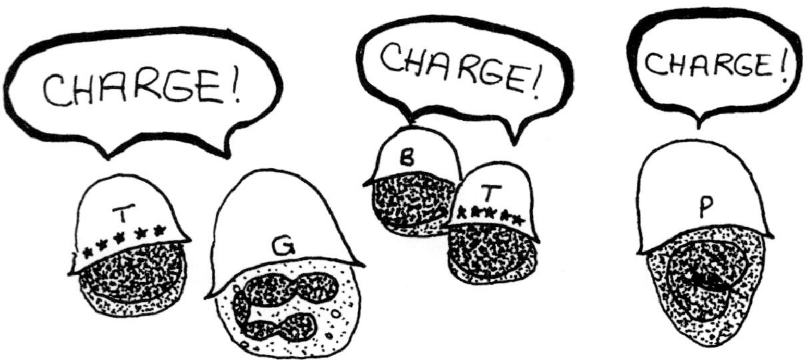

There are five main approaches
being *tested* now
in the use of immune boosters
to help treat HIV.

The first type of approach
is called "passive."
In this approach, you are given things
your own immune system would be making
if it was healthy.
The passive approach is now being *tested* in children,
using IVIG (see page 89).
IVIG uses antibodies from other people
to help you fight infections.
IVIG is given IV, either in the clinic or at home.
It takes about 4 hours for it to all get into your body,
so you might want to have a book to look at
or a T.V. to watch
while you wait.

Side effects that IVIG can cause are:

1. a sick feeling
2. fever and chills
3. headache
4. nausea and vomiting
5. chest or back pain
6. severe allergic reaction

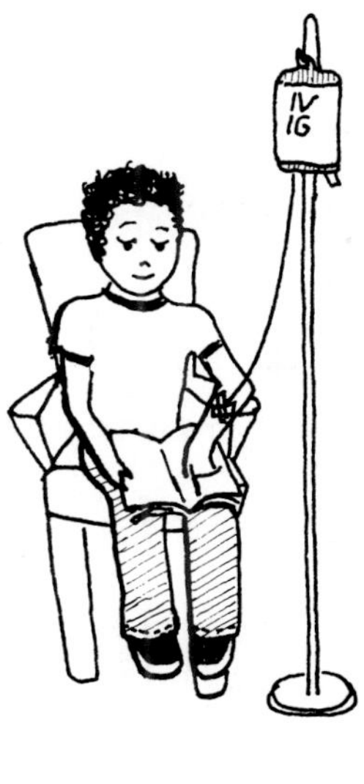

The second approach is both "active" and "specific,"
because your own immune system does most of the work,
and it's aimed at helping it fight HIV itself.
The best example of this is vaccines,
sort of like the ones you got when you were little.
What was in the vaccines
(the stuff that was in the shots)
were the antigens from germs that cause certain diseases.
These germ antigens are very different from yours.
When your immune system saw those germ antigens,
it went to work to make antibodies
and cells that could destroy these germs.
If you are ever exposed to these diseases again,
your immune system is ready to defend you.

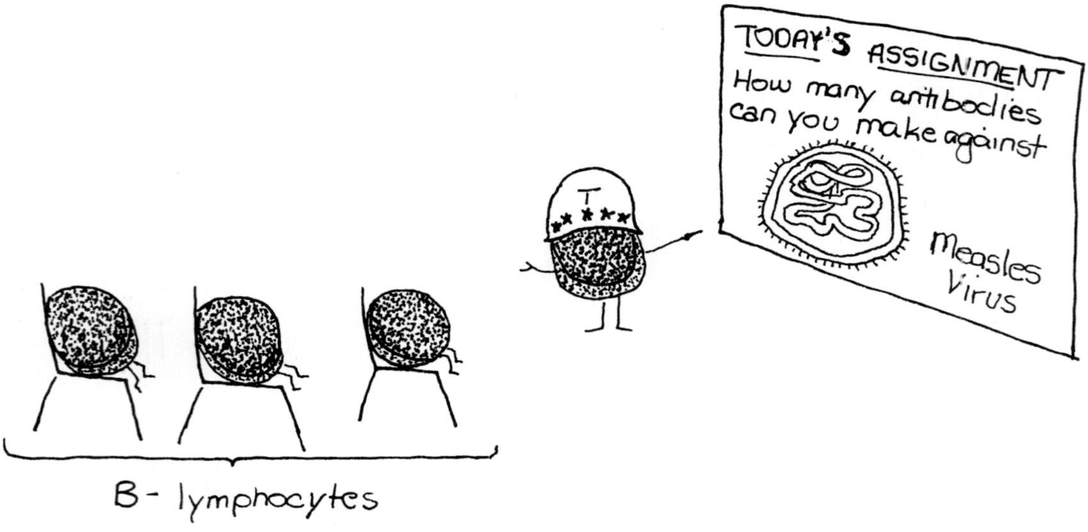
TODAY'S ASSIGNMENT
How many antibodies can you make against
Measles Virus
T
B- lymphocytes

Several vaccines are in development now
to be used to prevent HIV infection in uninfected people
or to stop HIV infection from getting worse
in people already infected.
At this time, there are several vaccines
that may work against HIV
that are now being *tested* in people.
Most of them are in the very early stages
and are just being tested to see
if they are safe to use in HIV-infected people.
A couple are now known to be safe,
so they are being tested to see if they can
slow down or stop HIV infection
by making the infected person's immune system
more active at getting rid of HIV and the cells it infects.
If these vaccines prove safe and effective,
they will be tested to see if they can prevent people
from getting infected with HIV in the first place.
But all of this is going to take a very long time.

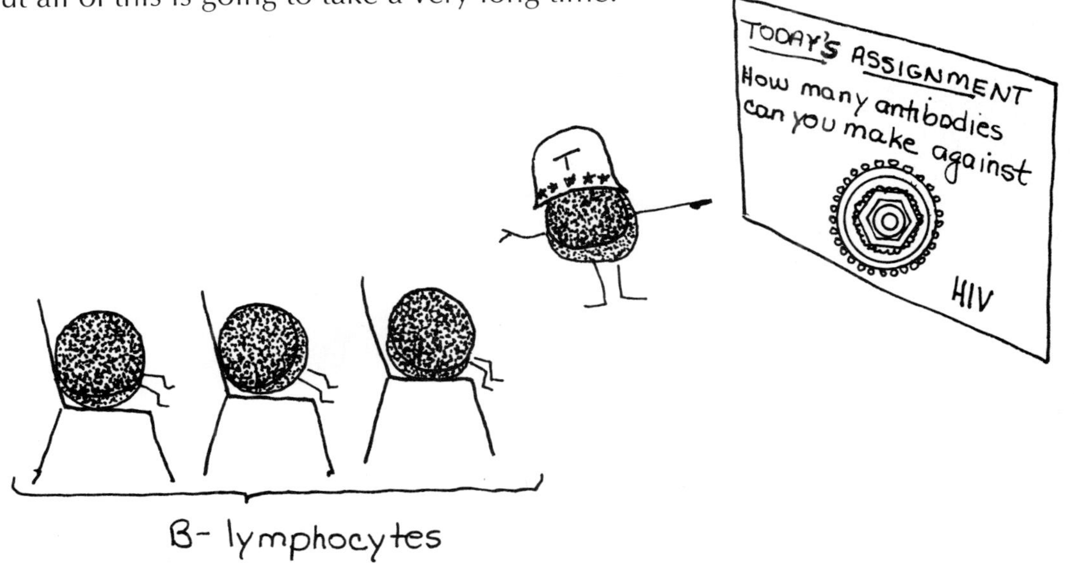
TODAY'S ASSIGNMENT
How many antibodies can you make against
HIV
T
B- lymphocytes

The third approach

is also active, but it's not specific.

This approach uses medicines that have been found

to make your whole immune system

more excited about doing its job.

It's kind of like the way you might feel

before you do something that is both important

and a little bit scary—

like running in a race.

All of you is just more alert and excited at those times,

and often, you find that you can do what you have to do

a little better than you thought you could.

This approach helps your immune system

do a better job at fighting all kinds of strange antigens,

not just HIV and its antigens.

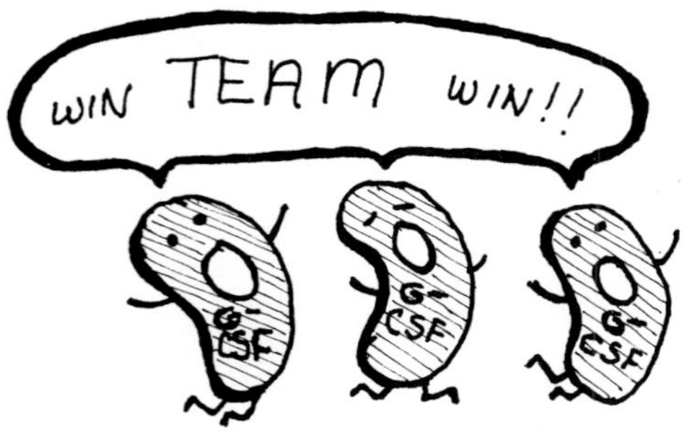

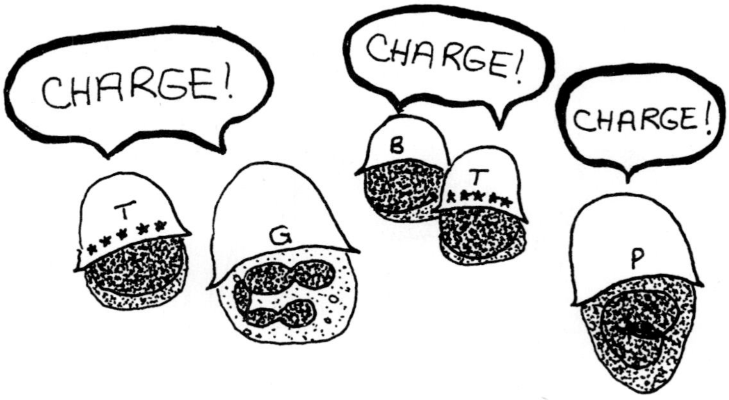

A substance that uses this approach is now being *tested* in children.
The substance is called G-CSF, which is short for **G**ranulocyte - **C**olony **S**timulating **F**actor.
It is given as a shot just under the skin (SC or Sub-Q).

Side effects that G-CSF can cause are:

1. mild fever
2. muscle, bone or joint aches and pains
3. headache
4. nausea
5. high white cell count (see page 75)
6. rash
7. swelling
8. diarrhea

Other medicines that may not get along with G-CSF are:
TMP/SMX, pentamidine, amphotericin B, flucytosine or interferons.

A medicine that may work better with G-CSF is AZT.

Other medicines that excite the immune system and are now being *tested* in adults include:
Ampligen, AS-101, thymopentin, lentinan, inosine pranobex, disulfiram, Imreg-1 and Imreg-2.

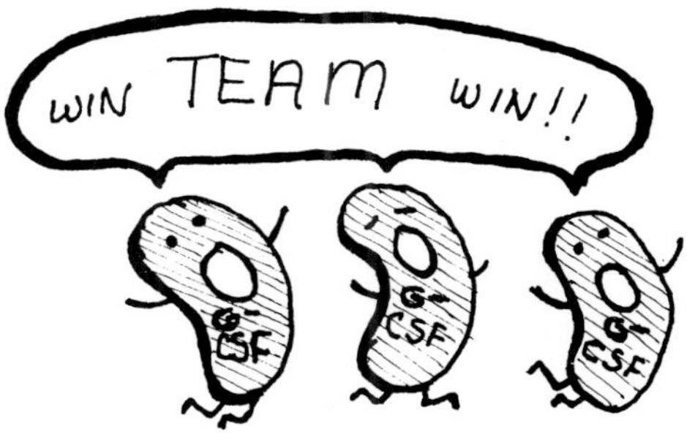

The fourth approach is called "adoptive."
As you know, helper T-cells not only fight germs,
they also give a lot of orders
to the other cells in the immune system
to help them do their jobs better.
When helper T-cells give orders,
they don't shout them with words
as people do.
They give orders by producing certain chemicals
called cytokines
that tell the other cells what to do.
A number of these cytokines are now being *tested*
in adults with HIV infection
to see if the rest of the immune system can work better
if someone just tells them what to do.
Cytokines that are now being tested in adults are:
tumor necrosis factor (TNF), interleukin-2 (IL-2),
and a whole bunch of interferons
(alpha interferon, interferon alfa-2a,
interferon alfa-2b, interferon alfa-nl,
interferon beta, and interferon gamma).
These chemical "orders" are being tested alone
and in combination with AZT and other medicines
to treat HIV infection.
This approach makes a lot of sense,
but no one really knows how well it will work.

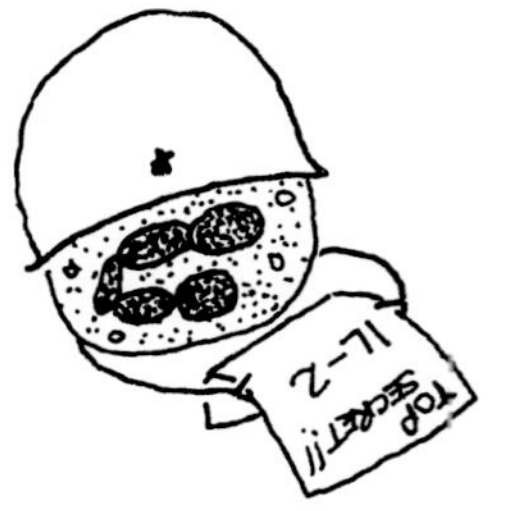

A fifth approach that has been *tried* in a few adults
but not yet in children
is bone marrow transplants.
All the cells of the immune system are born in the bone marrow,
the squishy part inside the hard part of bones.
Bone marrow transplants have been used
to treat people with certain kinds of blood cancers.
They are dangerous procedures,
but they can cure people with blood cancers.
A bone marrow transplant works
by giving a person a whole new immune system.
If a way could be found to kill all the HIV
hiding in phagocytes, brain cells and other organs—
as well as in the helper T-cells—
then it might make sense to use bone marrow transplants
to give people with HIV new immune systems—
immune systems that are not infected with HIV.
But, until a way can be found
to kill every HIV-infected cell in a person's body,
bone marrow transplants will be only a dream.

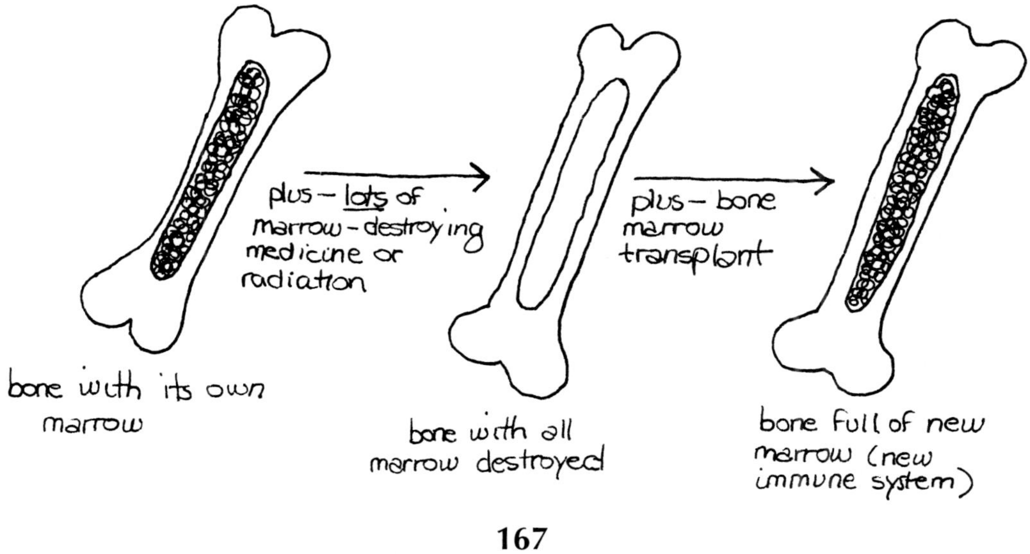

Supportive Therapy

Supportive therapy is all the things
you and your doctors will do
to treat the complications of HIV
and keep you feeling as good as possible.
Because so many things can happen with HIV,
this section on supportive therapy
can't include everything that might happen to you.
But some things happen often enough with HIV
that we thought you should know about them.

This section will be divided into two parts.
The first part will be about
the different things doctors do
to *diagnose*—or figure out—
what kinds of problems you are having.
The second part will be about
the different things doctors do
and the medicines they use
to *treat* those problems.

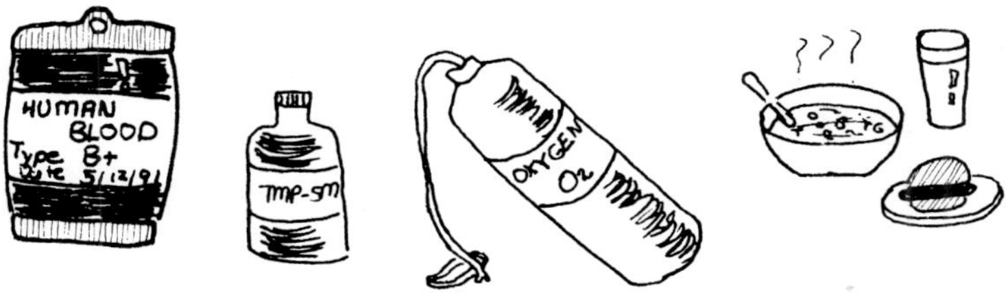

Diagnosing HIV Complications

You already know a lot
about how doctors diagnose things.
You know about the blood tests used
to diagnose, or figure out, if a person has HIV.
You know about blood tests used
to diagnose things like anemia and thrombocytopenia.
You know about how doctors figure out
what germ is causing an infection
by getting a sample of the infected part
(like blood or urine or saliva)
and then growing the germs outside the body
in a growth medium, or culture.
In addition to all these things,
there are some special things doctors do
to diagnose infections and other problems.
The most common ones will be described here.

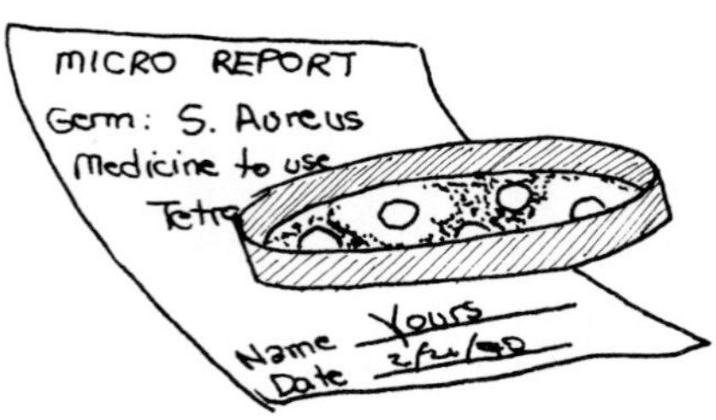

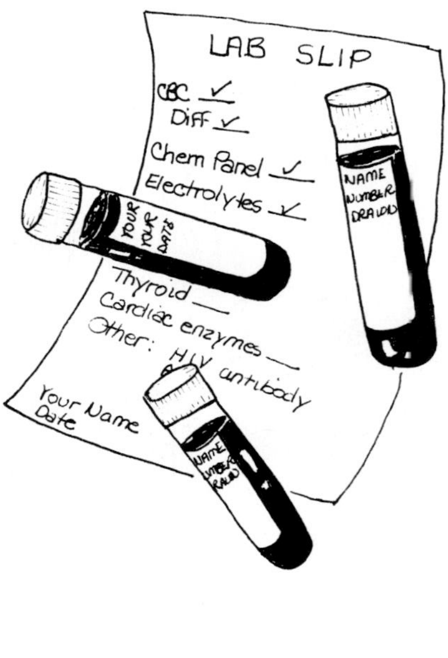

1. Biopsies

When your doctor thinks you have an infection
in a part of your body that is under your skin
but not in your blood,
the doctor may want to do a biopsy.
A biopsy just means getting a piece of the infected part
so that it can be looked at under a microscope
and the germs in it can be cultured.
Doctors have figured out ways
to help it not hurt you too much
when they do biopsies.
They do this by using something called anesthesia,
which is a word that means "no pain."
There are two kinds of anesthesia.
One kind is local anesthesia.
In this kind, special numbing medicine is used
that puts the nerves to sleep
near where the doctor will work
so you won't feel much besides a little pressure.
The other kind is called general anesthesia.
In this kind, *you* are put to sleep
so you won't feel anything at all until you wake up.
Because we can't guess what kinds of biopsies
you might need,
we're going to describe only two of them here—
one that is done with local anesthesia
and one that is done with general anesthesia.

Bone Marrow Biopsy

A bone marrow biopsy is an example
of a biopsy that is done with a local anesthesia.
This procedure isn't done often in HIV,
but it might be done if your doctor is worried
about your blood counts being too low or too high.
The bone marrow biopsy is also an example
of a kind of biopsy called a "needle biopsy,"
which can be done on other organs as well.

Bone marrow, as you already know,
is inside your bones.
To get a piece of it,
your doctor will put a needle into a bone
that is close to your skin—
like your hip bone or breast bone
or your shin bone if you're a tiny baby.

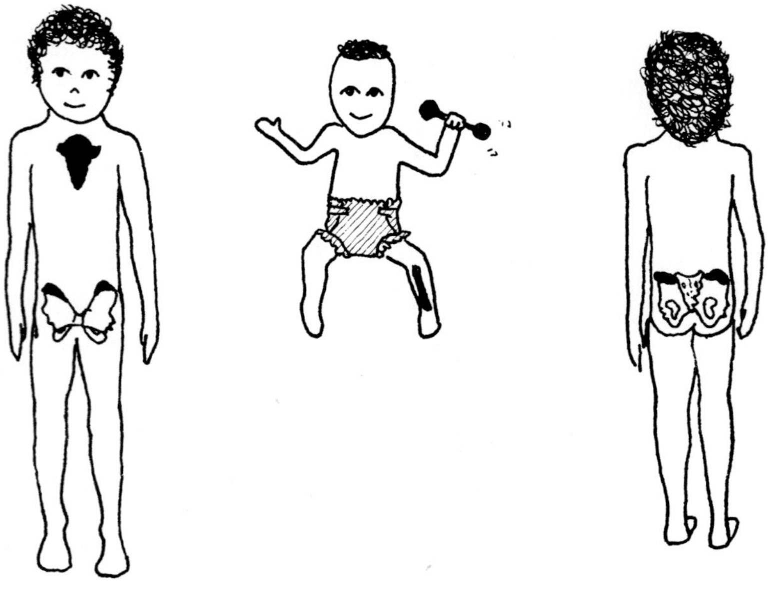

When you go for your bone marrow biopsy,
you will be asked to lie down on your tummy on a table.
Your pants and underpants will be pulled down a little
so that the doctor has room to work.
The doctor will examine your back.
Then the doctor will put on rubber gloves
and wipe your hip with cold stuff that kills germs
(an antiseptic).
Then he or she will put clean cloth or paper towels on you,
leaving only a little bit of your skin showing.
All of these things are done to protect you.
There are germs on your skin and on the doctor's skin, too.
No one wants those germs to get inside of you,
and gloves, towels and antiseptics keep germs away.
The needles that will be used are sterilized,
which means that they don't have any germs on them.
Nothing will touch you that isn't clean.

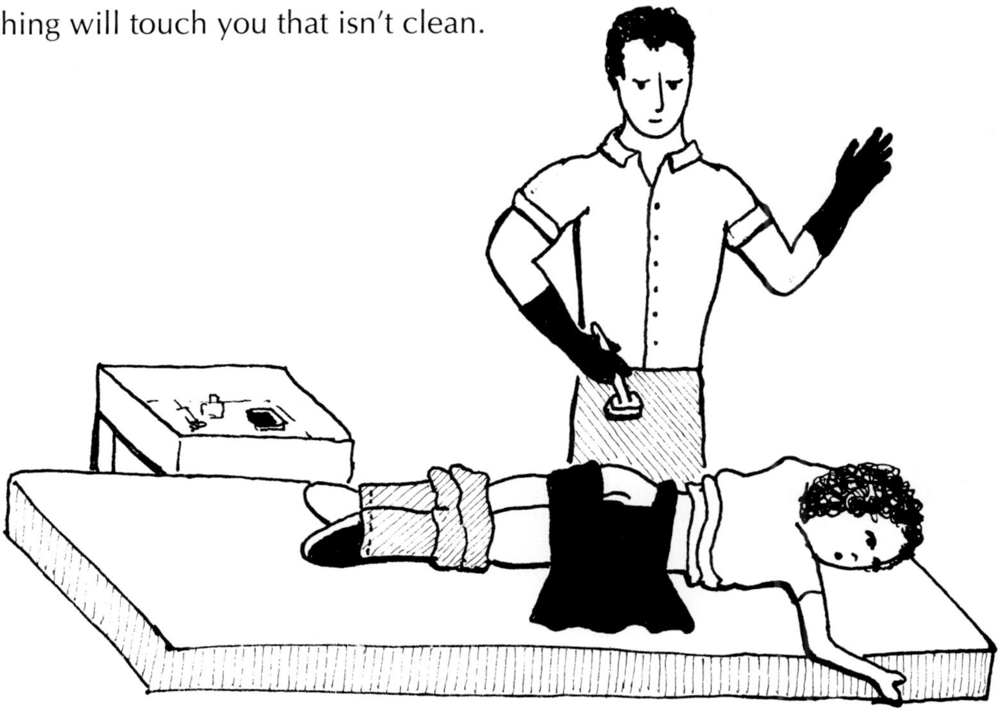

Now that you are prepared ("prepped"),
the doctor will give your back a shot of
numbing medicine (xylocaine).
The shot usually stings for a minute.
The xylocaine will be put where
the biopsy needle will go,
all the way down to the bone.

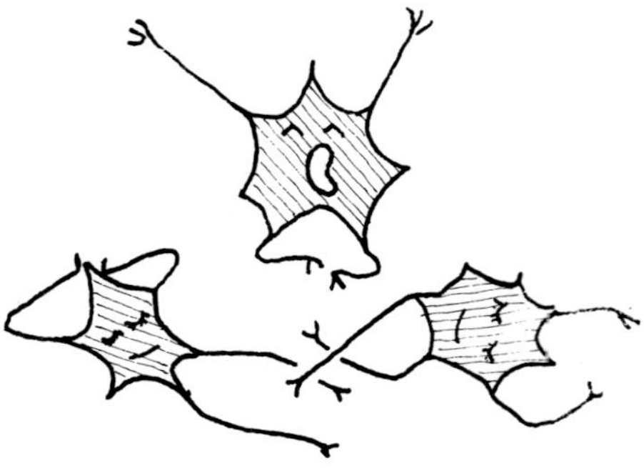

sleepy nerves

The medicine can't be put *into* the bone,
but since bones don't have any nerves,
you don't feel pain when the needle goes into your bones.
There are nerves in the stuff around bones.
Xylocaine makes most of these nerves so sleepy
that they don't send pain messages to your brain.
You will feel pain at the exact moment the needle
goes into your bone
because the outside lining of the bone is so full of nerves
that they can't all be put to sleep.
But the pain will be only at that exact moment
and only last—a moment.
When the medication is all in,
which only takes about a minute,
the doctor may wait a little while
to let the medicine put your nerves to sleep.
It usually works pretty fast.
While waiting, the doctor may examine your back again.

The doctor might then use a tiny knife,
called a scalpel,
to make a teeny opening in your skin.
Then the doctor will take a special needle
and slide it past the sleepy nerves and stuff
into your bone marrow.
The needle actually has two parts—a hollow outside tube
with a solid inside plug
so it's strong enough to go into a bone.
When the needle is in, the doctor will pull out the plug
and leave the hollow tube in place.
Then the doctor will push the hollow part in
just a little farther
until he or she thinks there's a piece of marrow in it.
Then the doctor pulls out the needle
and uses the plug part to push out the bone marrow piece
to be sure he or she got enough.
If it's a good sample, you're all done.
If not, the doctor may have to try again.
But don't worry—your nerves are still asleep
and it won't take much longer.

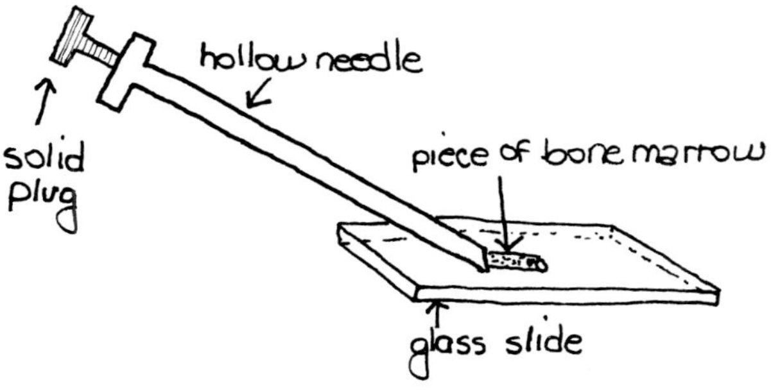

When the doctor has finished,
you just have to wait a few minutes
until you stop bleeding
(you won't bleed very much).
Then you'll get a bandage put on,
and you're all finished.
By the way, the bandage should stay on for a whole day.

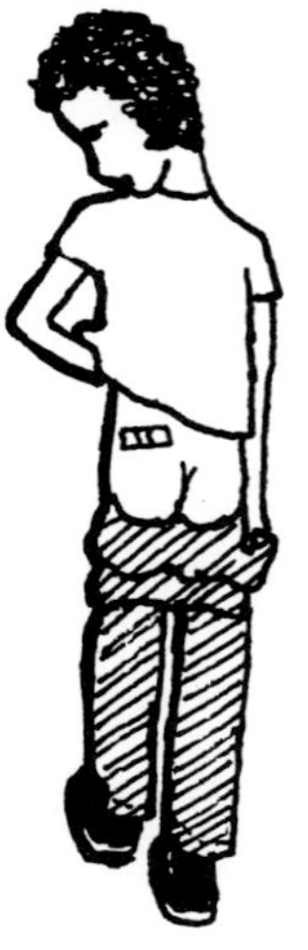

All biopsies done with local anesthesia
happen something like this.
Biopsy needles aren't always used,
sometimes scalpels are instead.
Sometimes you may need a few stitches
to close the opening made in your skin
(stitches are kind of like sewing—
only instead of sewing two pieces of cloth together,
stitches sew two pieces of skin together).
It all depends on what part of you
the doctor needs to biopsy.
The nice thing about biopsies done with local anesthesia
is that you're ready to go home right after.
The doctor can't go home, though.
He or she has to look at the biopsy
under a microscope.
If you have a biopsy,
ask your doctor to show it to you with the microscope.
You won't think it looks much like you—
but you'll probably think it's pretty.

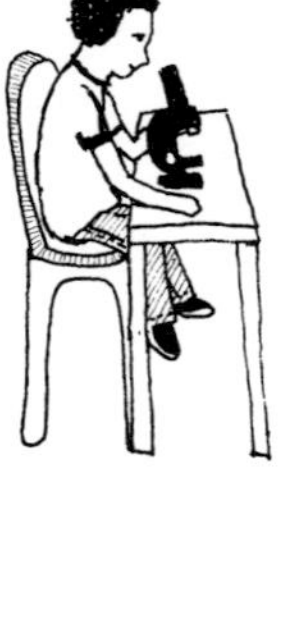

Open Lung Biopsy

When a person with HIV gets pneumonia,
or some kind of lung infection,
doctors can't tell by examining them
if it's PCP or LIP.
They can't tell by looking at X-rays, either
(X-rays are pictures of your insides).
So, in order to give you the right treatment
they may need to do an open lung biopsy.
An open lung biopsy is an operation.
It is done in an operating room
by a special kind of doctor called a surgeon.
Open lung biopsies can't be done
with local anesthesia,
because there's no way to get all the nerves
that will be bothered by the procedure asleep.
So, instead, *you* are put to sleep
using a general anesthesia.

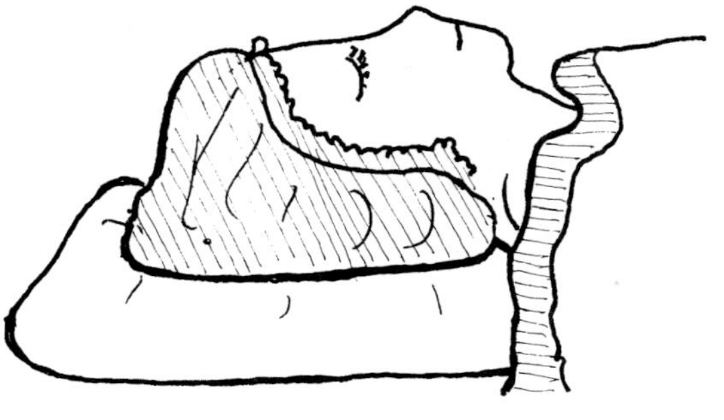

Before you go to sleep, you'll be put on a weird, hard bed,
and a funny paper shower cap will be put on your head.
You'll be given some medicines that will help you relax
and that will also make your mouth feel very dry.
The person in charge of your anesthesia,
who might be a doctor or a nurse,
will put an IV in your arm
which is how you'll get the medicine
that will make you sleep.
You'll also notice that everyone is wearing
strange, bluish-greenish clothes
that kind of look like pajamas and bathrobes.
They'll also be wearing funny paper slippers, masks and gloves,
and shower caps like yours.
All of these things are worn
to keep the germs on the doctors and nurses
from getting into you during the operation.

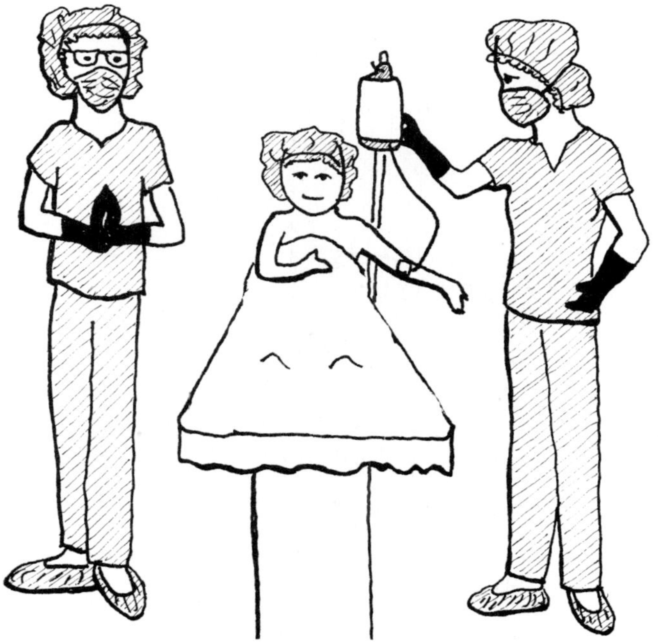

Once you are sound asleep,
the surgeon will make a cut
in the skin on the front of your chest
between two of your ribs.
This cut will be made deeper
until the doctor sees your lung.
Then, a small piece of your lung will be removed.
The edges of the lung will be stitched back together
so it won't leak air afterwards.
Then your muscles and skin
will be stitched back together, too.
The only stitches you'll see
when you wake up
will be the ones in your skin.
You may also see a small, clear plastic tube
coming out of the place where the surgeon worked.
This is called a chest tube.
Sometimes, after lung operations,
liquids leak from the nearby cells.
A chest tube is a way for these liquids
to get out of your body
instead of squishing your lungs.
Both the chest tube and the stitches
will come out in a few days.

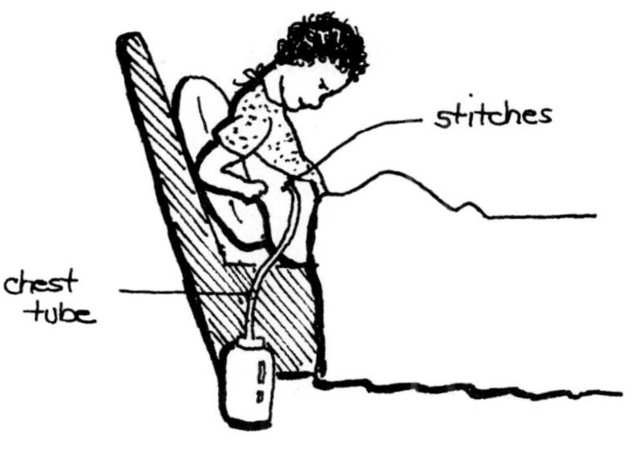

After the open lung biopsy is finished,
you'll be taken to a place called a recovery room,
which is also often a Pediatric Intensive Care Unit
(or "Peds. I.C.U.").
That's where you'll wake up—
so don't be surprised to be in a different place
than you were when you fell asleep.
Nurses there will do things like take your pulse,
check your blood pressure,
and make sure your IV is working well.
(You usually have to have an IV going
for a few days after most operations.)
They will also check your chest tube, if you have one.
Almost everyone, when they wake up from surgery,
finds that they have funny little tubes in their nose
to give them oxygen.
Because your operation was on your lungs,
you may find yourself attached
to a machine called a ventilator.
The machine helps you breathe
by pushing air in and pulling it out
through a tube that goes from your mouth
to the tubes in your respiratory system.
Usually, your lungs start working again pretty quick,
and you'll only be on the ventilator a short time.

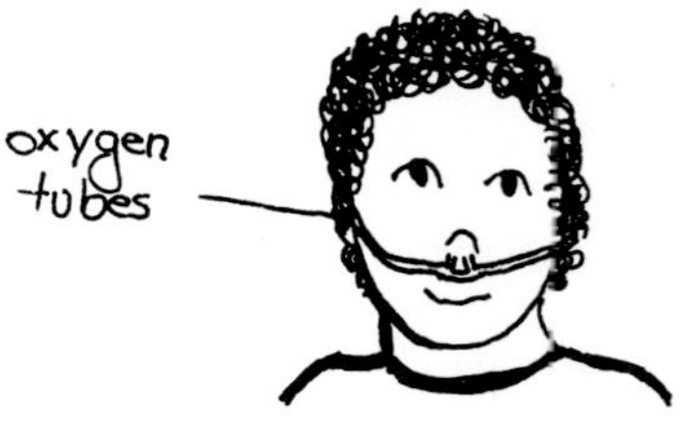

When your doctors and nurses
think you're doing well enough,
the tubes will be taken out of you,
and you'll be taken to another room in the hospital
where you'll be staying for a few days.
During this time, your doctors will figure out
if you have PCP or LIP,
and you will start getting medicines for this.
You may still need to get oxygen (see pages 236-237).
The place on your chest where the operation was done
will probably be sore for a while.
You'll be given medicines to help you feel more comfortable.
If you're hurting a lot,
don't be afraid to tell your doctor and nurses
so they can give you stronger medicine for the pain.
And, once you're in your own room,
you can have lots of visitors.

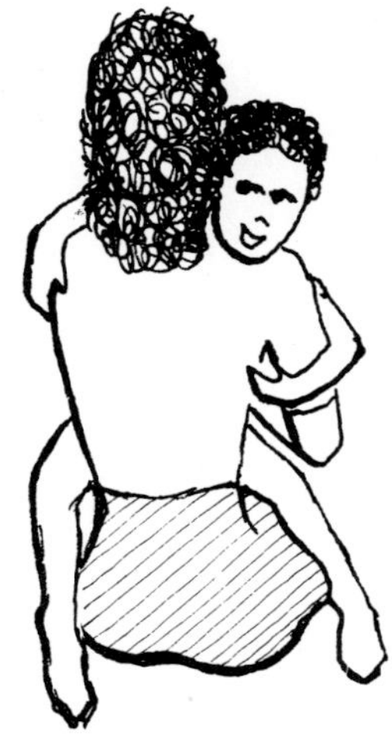

Most procedures done using general anesthesia
happen something like this one,
whether it's for a biopsy or something else.
General anesthesia is great
because you don't feel anything at all
until after the operation is all finished.
One thing that's not so great about it, though,
is it can make you feel kind of mixed up afterwards,
and it can make some people feel sick to their stomachs.
You might also have a sore throat
from the tube that was used to help you breathe
during the operation.
These feelings go away quickly.

Another thing about operations
is that kids get better from them
a lot faster than grownups do.
So if you have to have an operation,
you and your parents or caretakers
can be pretty sure
that you'll be feeling much better
in a few days.

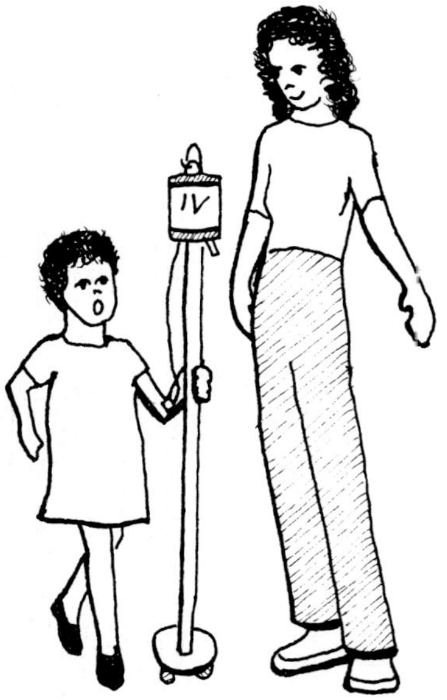

2. Bronchial Alveolar Lavage

A procedure that a few doctors are using
to decide whether you have PCP or LIP
is called bronchial alveolar lavage or BAL.
This can be done under either local or general anesthesia,
depending on what your doctor thinks is best for you.
In this procedure, you don't get cut anywhere,
and you don't need stitches.
Before BAL is done, you'll be given medicines
to relax you and that will make your mouth feel dry.
BAL is done by putting a skinny tube
called a bronchoscope
deep down into the tubes of your respiratory system.

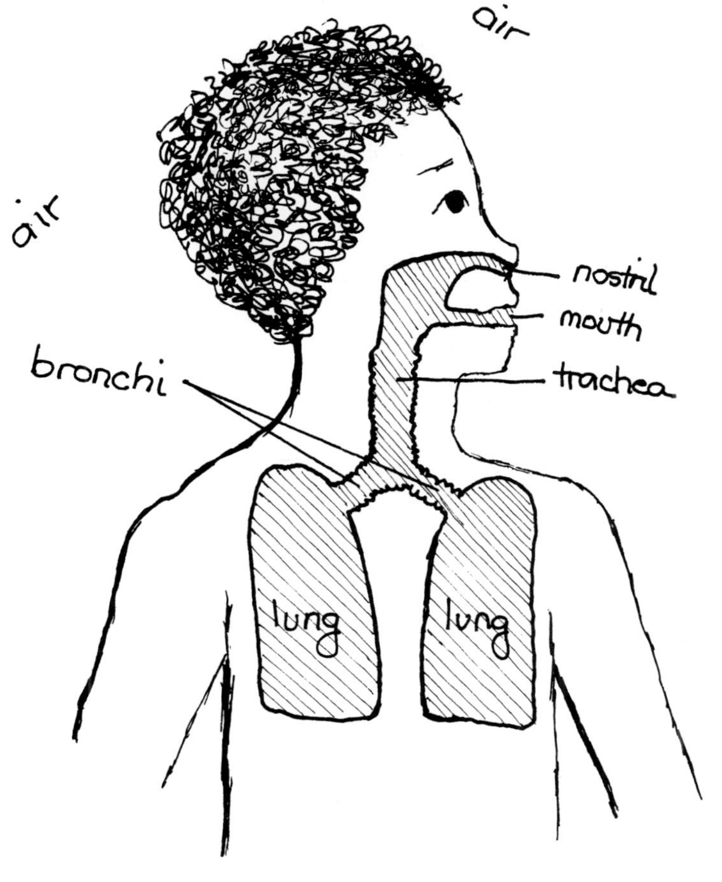

Then, samples of your mucus—
the fluid that lines the respiratory system—
are taken out through the bronchoscope,
and then the bronchoscope is taken out.
The samples of your mucus are looked at under microscopes
and put into growth mediums to see if PCP grows.
This procedure is often done in adults,
and it is being used more and more often in children.
The good thing about it is that
it's not as hard on you as having an open lung biopsy.
The bad thing is that if no germs grow in the culture,
you might still have to have an open lung biopsy anyway.

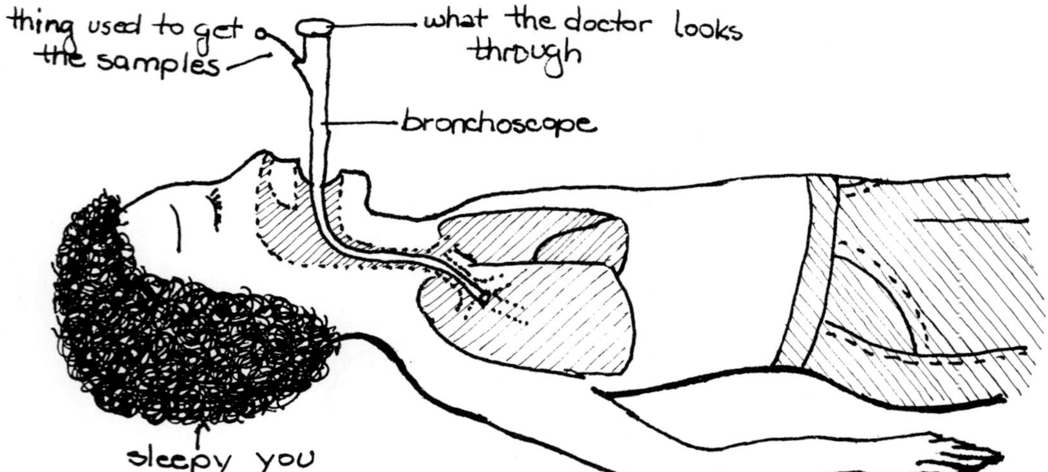

3. CT Scans and MRI

Sometimes doctors need to "see" inside your body
in order to figure out what's troubling you.
For a long time, doctors have used X-rays to do this.
But while X-rays are great at showing
problems with things like bones or teeth,
they're often not so great at showing problems
with softer organs in your body.
So, doctors have figured out ways
to take good pictures of your softer parts.
CT (or "CAT") scans and MRI scans
are how they do this.
The good thing about these procedures
is that they don't hurt at all.
The bad thing about them
is that they take a long time,
they are very boring,
you have to hold very still,
and you have to be put inside a machine for a while.

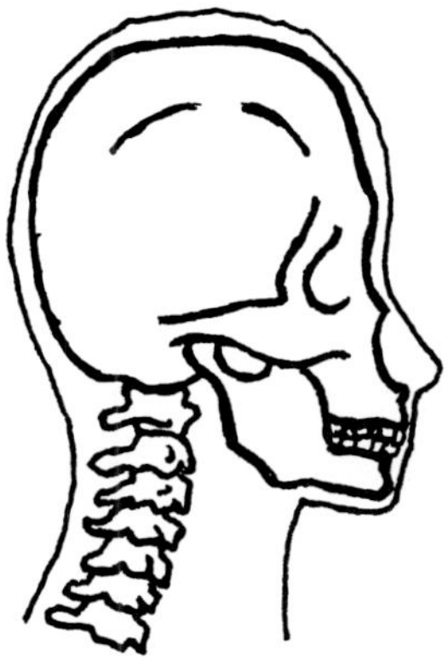

X-Rays show bones

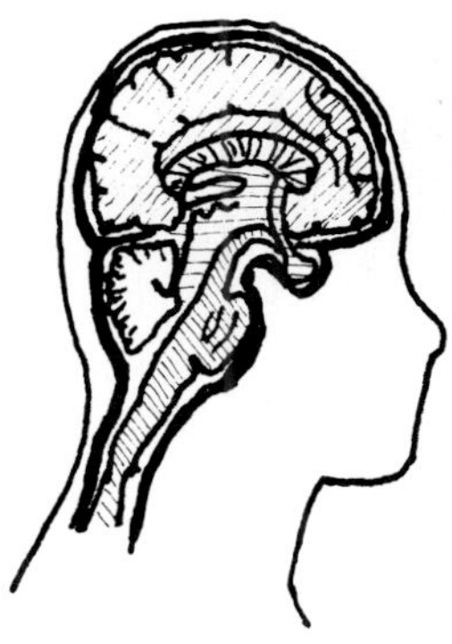

CT Scans and MRI scans show soft parts

The machine that you will be put into
is very, very big.
It's so big that it usually has its own room.
The machine has an opening in it
that's kind of like a tunnel,
and there is a hard table
that slides in and out of the tunnel.
When you are going to have a CT scan or an MRI,
you will lay down on this table,
and you and the table will slide into the tunnel.
That's all there is to it.
The big machine does the rest,
by taking a whole bunch of pictures
of the soft parts of your body
that your doctors want to see.

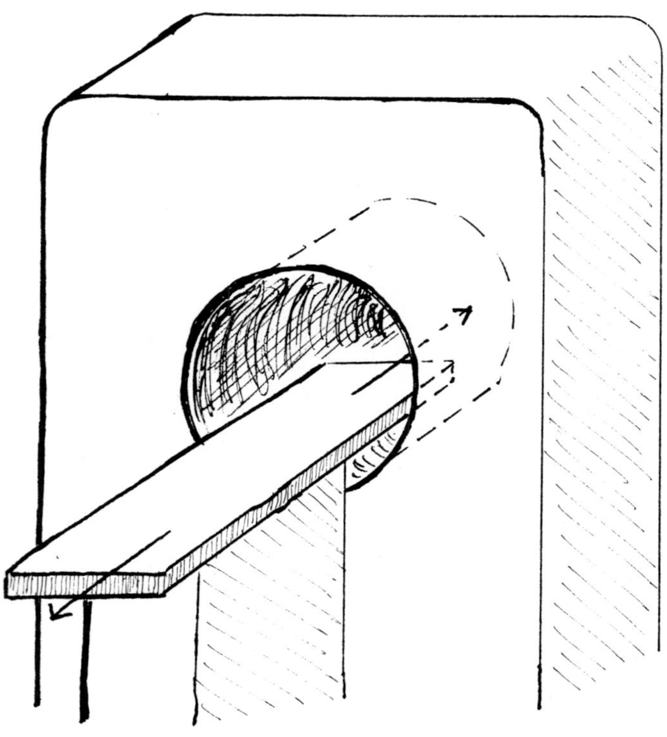

The thing is,

it takes a long time to take all these pictures.

You have to hold very still

while they're being taken.

And it gets kind of lonely there in the tunnel.

Even grownups don't like the lonely feeling

they can have while they're in the tunnel.

If you're having an MRI,

it can also be very noisy in the tunnel.

So, you and your doctors might decide

that it would be better if you were asleep

while having your CT scan or MRI.

That can help you hold still

and not be bored or lonely.

It all depends on how old you are

and how good you are at holding still

even when you're bored.

If you and your doctors decide it would be better

for you to be asleep,

you will be given a medicine called a sedative

which can be either a pill or an IV.

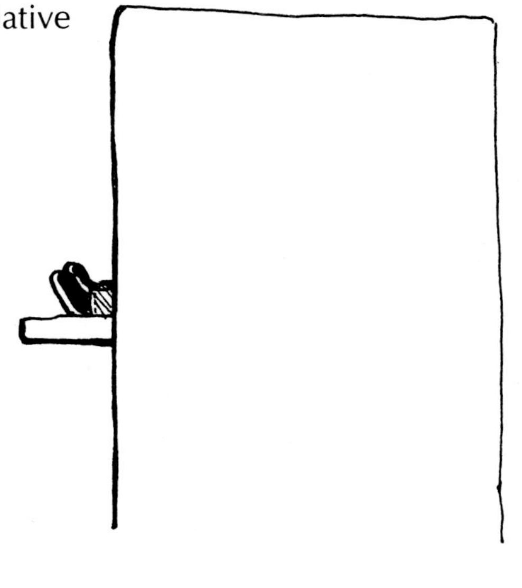

Once the machine is done
taking all those pictures,
you're all finished, too.
You can get up and go home
or do whatever else you were going to do that day.
One thing you might want to do
is to ask the doctor to show you the pictures sometime.
They're pretty interesting.
Ask the doctor what the different things
in the pictures are.
All those things are just parts of you
that you would never get a chance to see
any other way.

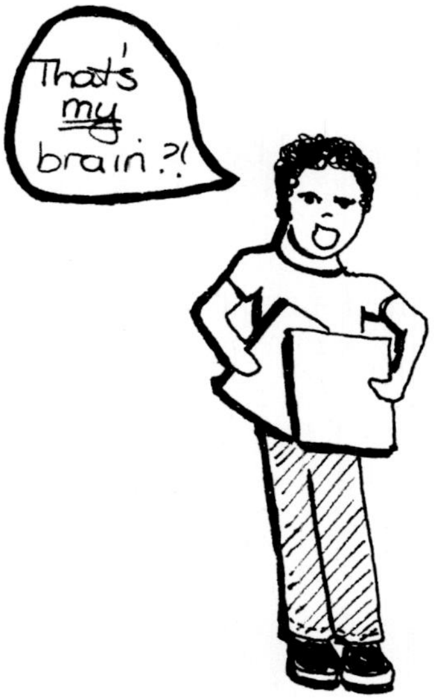

4. *Spinal Taps*

If your doctor thinks you might have
an infection of either your brain
or the lining around it
(called the meninges),
he or she may want you to have a spinal tap.
A spinal tap,
which is also called a lumbar puncture (LP),
is a way that your doctor can get a sample
of the fluid (called CSF)
that is inside the brain and spinal cord.
By doing tests on the CSF
and by putting some of it in a growth medium,
the doctors can tell if you have an infection
and learn how to treat it.
Spinal taps can also be used
to put medicine into the CSF
if it can't get there any other way.

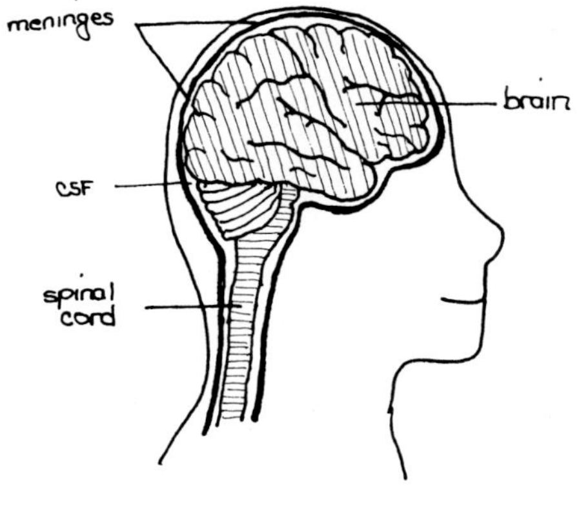

Spinal taps are done
either at the hospital or the clinic.
You have to lie down on your side on a table.
You will need to pull up your shirt
and lower your pants or skirt a little.
The doctor will ask you to curl up your body
by bringing your knees to your chest.
Your parent or caretaker
will probably help to hold you in this position.
That's because the more curled up you are,
and the stiller you are,
the easier it is for the doctor to work.
And that means that it won't hurt you very much.

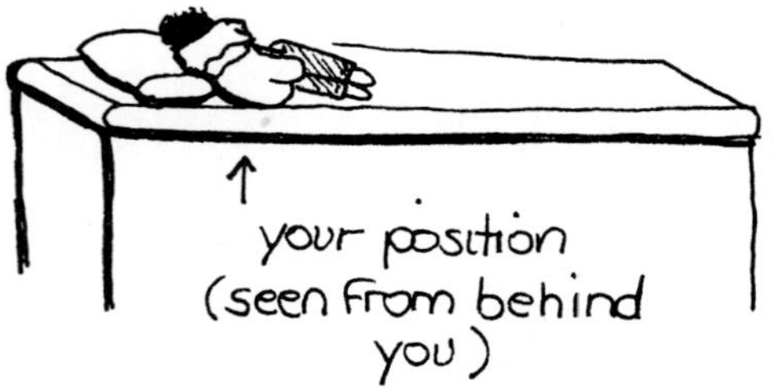

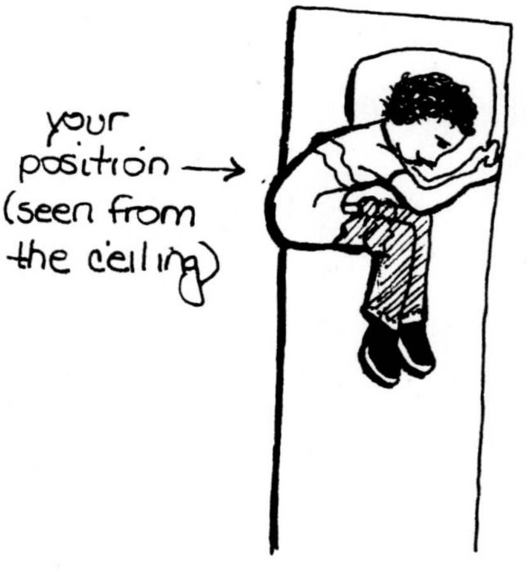

The doctor will stand behind you.
You will be prepared in about the same way
as for a bone marrow or other needle biopsy.
The doctor will wear gloves and put towels on you
and wipe off your back with an antiseptic to kill germs.
The doctor will feel your back
for the very best place to put the needle in.
Then you will be given a shot of numbing medicine
to make your nerves fall asleep.
This can burn and sting
but only for a few minutes.

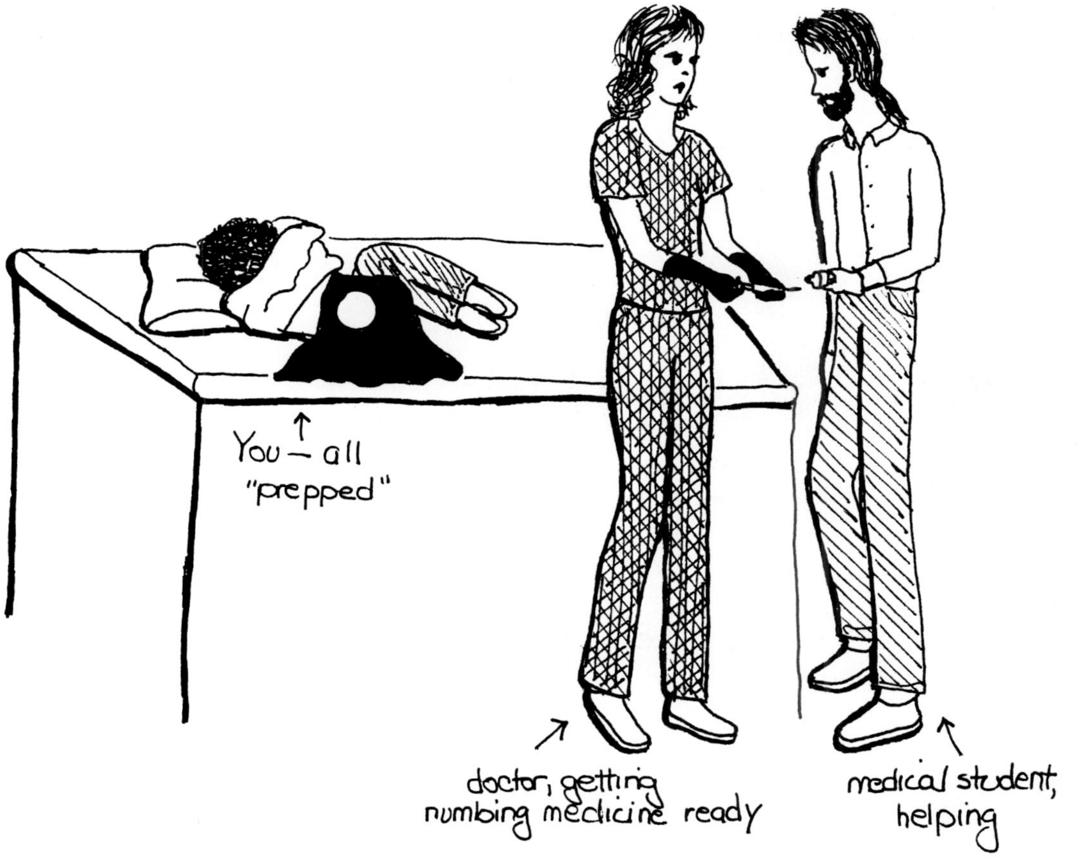

When your nerves have gotten very sleepy,
the doctor will take a special needle
(which has two parts, like the bone marrow needle)
and slide it past the sleepy nerves
through the meninges
into the space where the CSF is found.
The doctor can tell when he or she is in the right place
because CSF (which looks just like water)
will begin to drip out of the hollow needle.
After this, it shouldn't hurt at all
unless you move.
The doctor may then measure the pressure of the CSF
with a thing that looks like a big thermometer.

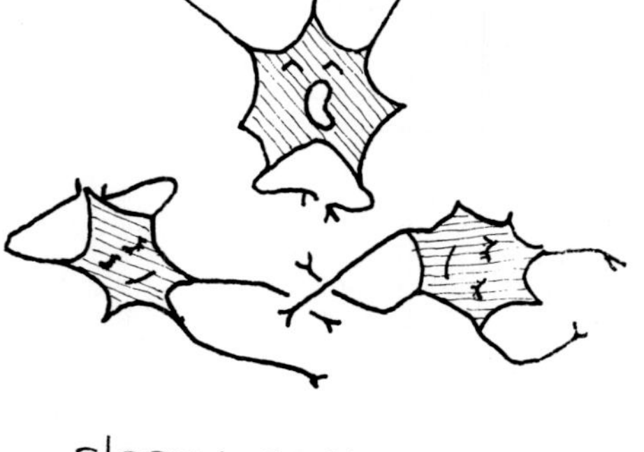

sleepy nerves

Then, the doctor will let some of the CSF
drip out into some test tubes,
which are little tubes like the ones
your blood is put into during blood tests.
After that, the doctor may measure
the CSF pressure again.
Then, the doctor will take the needle out.
You might feel a bandage being put on.
The doctor will want you to stay lying down
for about an hour after the spinal tap.
This is because some people get headaches
if they get up too soon after a spinal tap.
When your doctor thinks you're going to be all right,
you can get up and go.
But you might want to take it easy
the rest of the day,
just to be sure you don't get a headache.

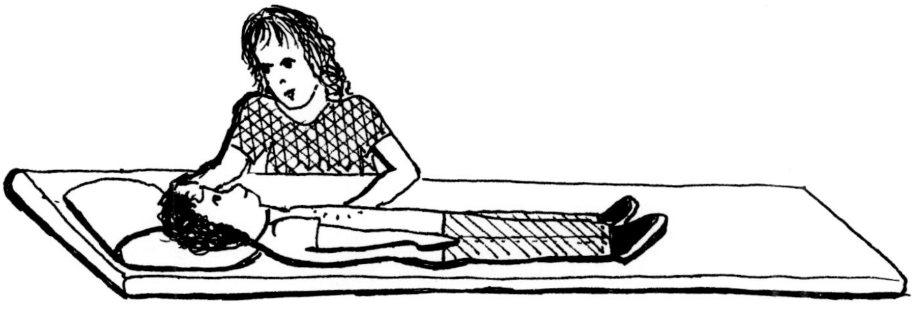

5. Other Procedures

This page is for you to use

to write down information about other procedures

your doctor wants you to have.

Treating HIV Complications

You already know a lot
about what doctors do
to treat the complications of HIV.
This section will just tell you more about it.
You will learn about many of the medicines
that are used to treat different kinds of infections
that children with HIV can get.
You will learn more about blood transfusions.
You will learn more about central lines.
You will learn more about oxygen.
You will learn more about pain management.
The writer of this book
couldn't know exactly what your treatment would be,
so she has included most of the medicines and procedures
that are commonly used.
At the end of this section,
there will be some blank pages for you to use
to write down things about other medicines
or other procedures
that are not talked about here.

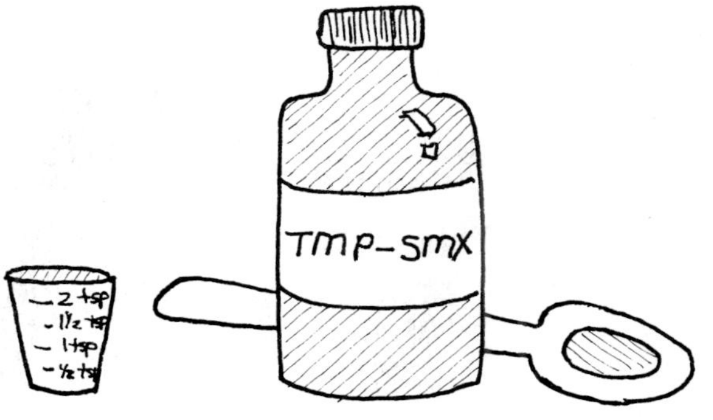

1. Anti-Infectives

Anti-infectives are medicines
that are used to treat infections.
Some are antibiotics, which are used to treat infections
caused by the group of germs called bacteria.
Some are antifungals, which are used to treat infections
caused by the group of germs called fungi.
Some are antiprotozoals, which are used to treat infections
caused by the group of germs called parasites.
Some are used to treat more than one kind of germ.
Each will be listed according to its most common use
in treating HIV-related infections.

As with antivirals, immune boosters,
and all other medicines,
anti-infectives can have side effects.
They can also react badly,
or be helped to work better,
by being combined with other medicines.
Unlike antivirals, though,
anti-infectives often cure the infection
that they are used to treat.

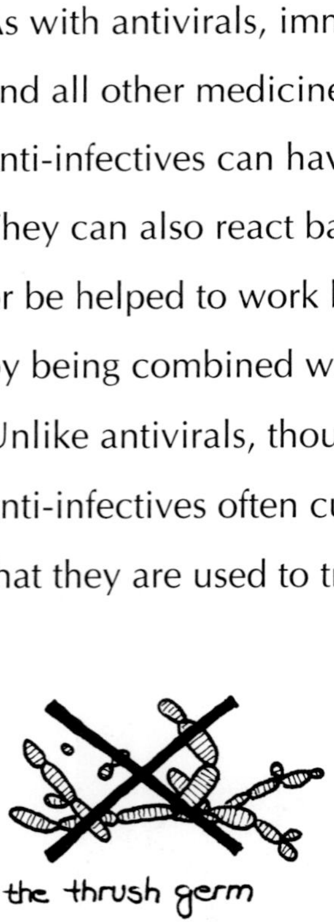

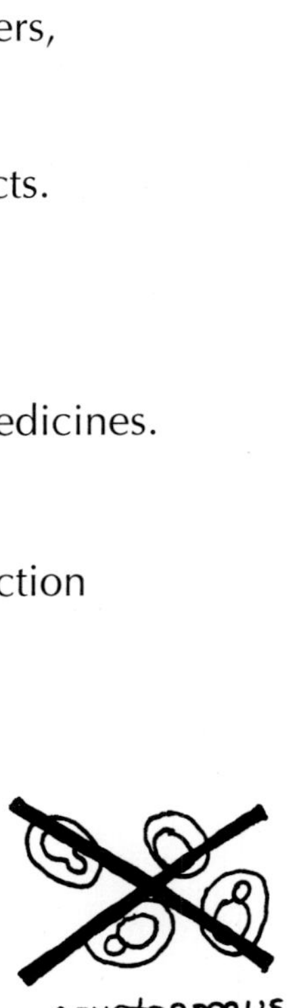

Amoxicillin

has a lot of other names.

It is an antibiotic, a kind of penicillin,

and is used to treat many kinds of infections

caused by bacteria in children and adults—

including children and adults with HIV.

It comes as a pill, a liquid, or drops for babies.

The liquid needs to be kept in the refrigerator.

It is usually given three or four times a day.

As with all antibiotics,

you should take it as long as your doctor tells you to,

even though you will feel better before that.

Most people, including children,

don't have trouble with side effects from amoxicillin,

unless they are allergic to penicillin—

and then they shouldn't take amoxicillin.

Side effects that amoxicillin can cause are:

1. diarrhea
2. rash
3. nausea and vomiting

A medicine that can help amoxicillin work better

is probenecid.

For this reason, they are often used together.

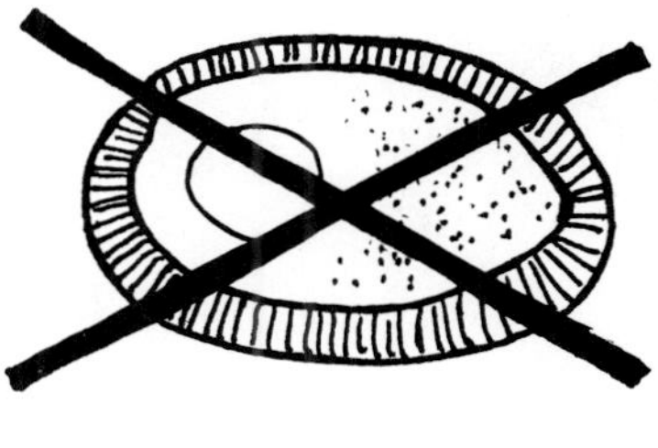

Ampicillin

has a lot of other names.

It is an antibiotic, a kind of penicillin,

and is used to treat many kinds of infections

caused by bacteria in children and adults—

including children and adults with HIV.

It comes as a pill or a liquid.

The liquid needs to be kept in the refrigerator.

It is usually given four times a day.

As with all antibiotics,

you should take it as long as your doctor tells you to,

even though you will feel better sooner.

Most people don't have much trouble

with side effects from ampicillin

unless they are allergic to penicillin—

and then they shouldn't take ampicillin.

Side effects that ampicillin can cause are:

1. sore tongue
2. diarrhea
3. rash
4. nausea and vomiting

A medicine that can help ampicillin work better

is probenecid.

For this reason, they are often used together.

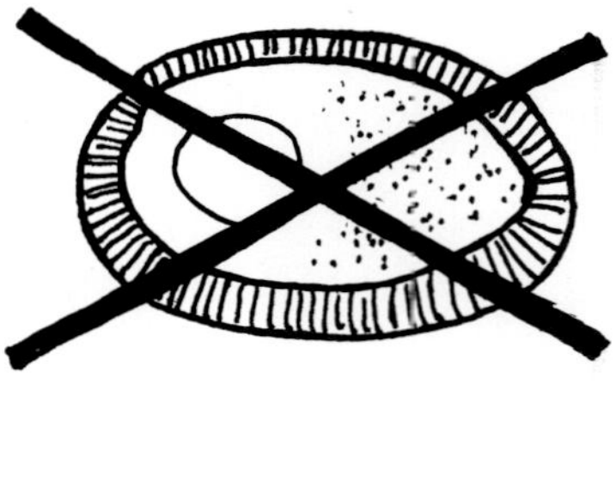

Ceftriaxone

is also called Rocephin.

It belongs to a group of antibiotics called cephalosporins.

It is used to treat many kinds of serious infections

caused by bacteria in children and adults—

including children and adults with HIV.

It is given IV or IM (a shot into a muscle),

once or twice a day for several days.

Most people do not have much trouble

with side effects from ceftriaxone

unless they are allergic to cephalosporins—

and then they shouldn't take ceftriaxone.

Side effects that ceftriaxone can cause are:

1. pain at the place it was injected
2. rash
3. diarrhea

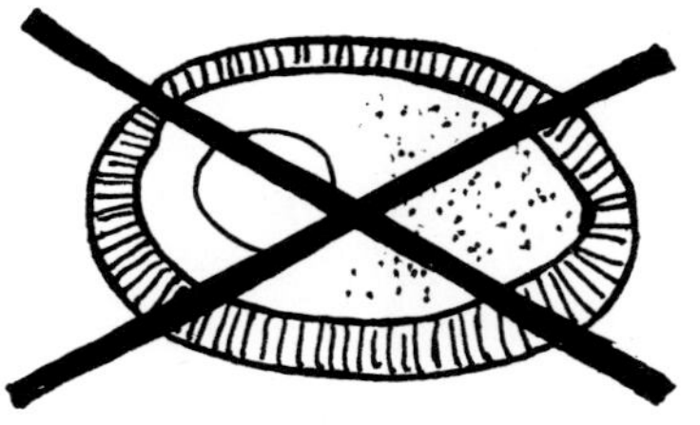

Clofazimine

is also called Lamprene.

It is an antibiotic that is used now and then

to treat infections caused by the group of bacteria

called mycobacteria,

especially leprosy and tuberculosis.

It is now being *tested* to prevent *M. avium* infections

in some people with HIV.

It comes as a pill

and should be taken with food.

It is taken once a day for a long time.

Side effects that clofazimine can cause are:

1. darkening of the skin
2. dry, scaly or itchy skin
3. stomachache
4. nausea and vomiting
5. diarrhea
6. dry, itchy or burny eyes

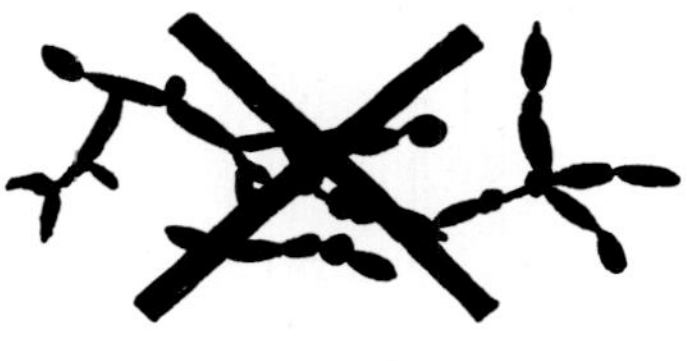

m. avium

Rifabutin

is also called Ansamycin.

It is an antibiotic that is sometimes used

to treat tuberculosis infections

when other antituberculosis medicines don't work.

It is being *tested* to prevent and treat

M. avium infections in people with HIV.

It comes as a pill.

There is no information about side effects

caused by rifabutin.

Medicines that can help rifabutin work better are:

ethambutol, ciprofloxacin, amikacin,

clofazimine, rifampin, and erythromycin.

All of these are also antibiotics,

and most are also used to treat tuberculosis.

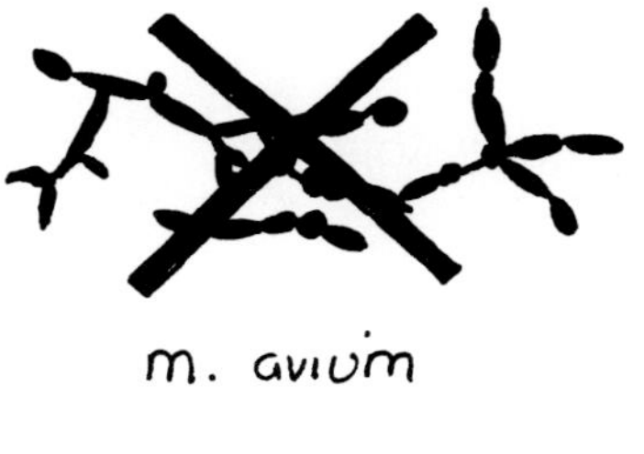

Amphotericin B

has many other names.

It is an antifungal medicine

and is used to treat serious fungal infections

in adults and children—

including adults and children with HIV.

It is given IV.

Side effects that amphotericin B can cause are:

1. fever and chills
2. muscle and joint pains
3. nausea and vomiting
4. diarrhea
5. anemia
6. kidney problems

A medicine that can help amphotericin B work better

and is sometimes given with it

is another antifungal called flucytosine (5-FC).

5-FC comes as a pill.

It has many side effects,

so the two have to be used carefully together.

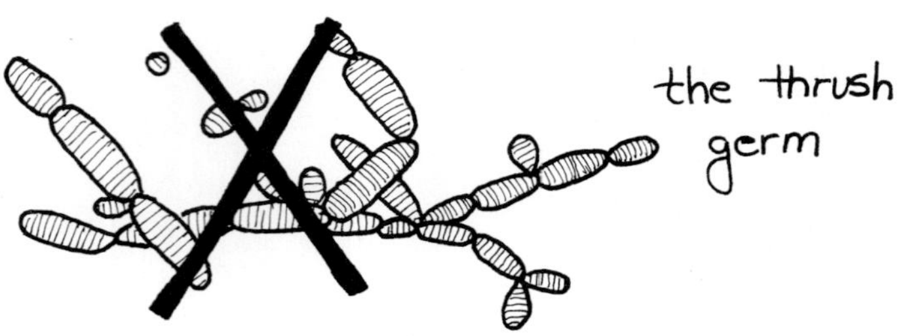

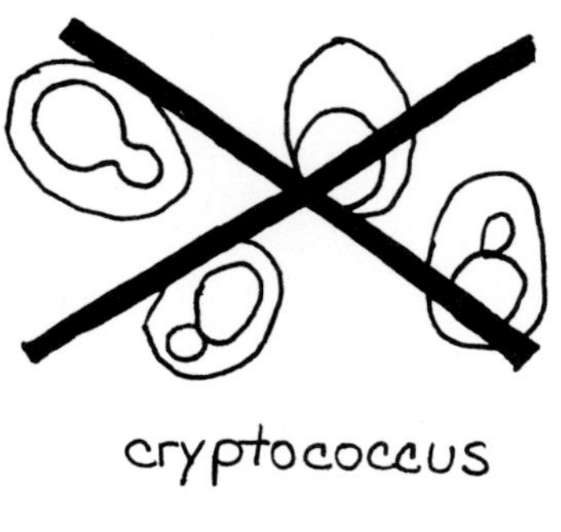

Ketoconazole

is also called Nizoral.

It is an antifungal that is used to treat

many kinds of fungal infections in adults and children—

including adults and children with HIV.

It comes as a pill or a cream

and can be used for a long time.

Side effects that ketoconazole can cause are:

1. dark-colored urine
2. light-colored bowel movements
3. a tired or weak feeling
4. stomachache
5. yellow eyes or skin

   (call your doctor if this happens)

Medicines that should not be taken with ketoconazole

are antacids.

A medicine that is a lot like ketoconazole

is another antifungal called itraconazole.

It is most often used to treat histoplasmosis.

It comes as a pill.

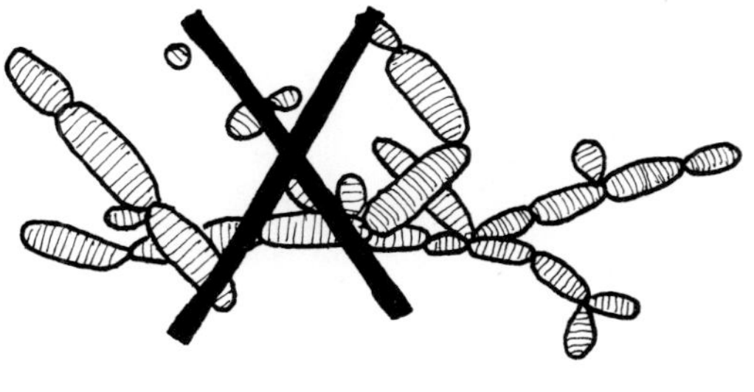

the thrush germ

Clotrimazole

has many other names.

It is an antifungal medicine

and is used to treat thrush

and other infections caused by the Candida fungus

in adults and children—

including adults and children with HIV.

It comes as a pill, a cream, or a lozenge.

A lozenge is kind of like a big cough drop

that you put into your mouth

and slowly suck on until it's all gone.

Most people don't have much trouble with side effects

from clotrimazole.

Side effects that clotrimazole can cause are:

1. stomachache
2. diarrhea
3. nausea and vomiting

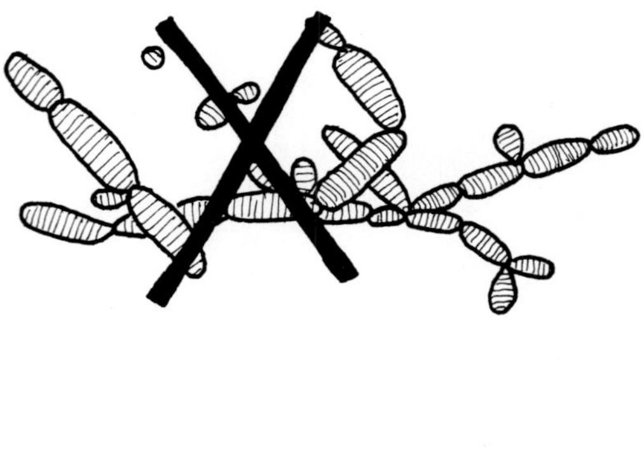

the thrush germ

Nystatin

has many other names.

It is an antifungal medicine

that is used to treat thrush

and other infections caused by the Candida fungus

in adults and children—

including adults and children with HIV.

It comes as a pill, a lozenge,

a cream, an ointment (a sticky cream),

and a liquid that you swish around in your mouth

before you swallow it.

It can be taken for a long time.

Almost no one ever has side effects from nystatin.

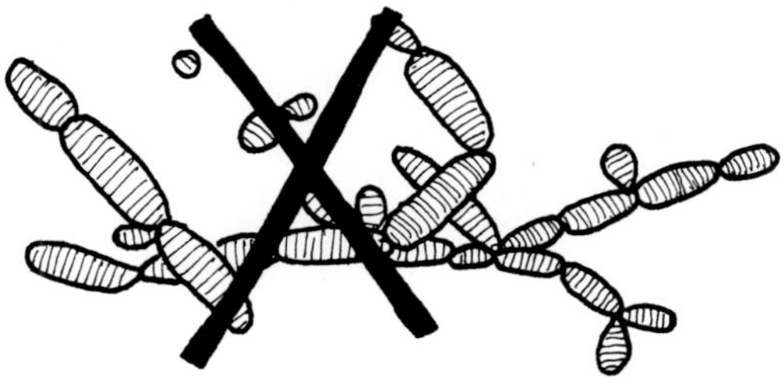

the thrush germ

Fluconazole

is also called Diflucan.

It is an antifungal medicine

that is used to treat infections caused by Candida

and brain infections caused by cryptococcus

in adults and children—

including adults and children with HIV.

It comes as a pill or IV

and can be given for a long time.

Side effects that fluconazole can cause are:

1. nausea
2. stomachache
3. headache
4. a slowed down feeling

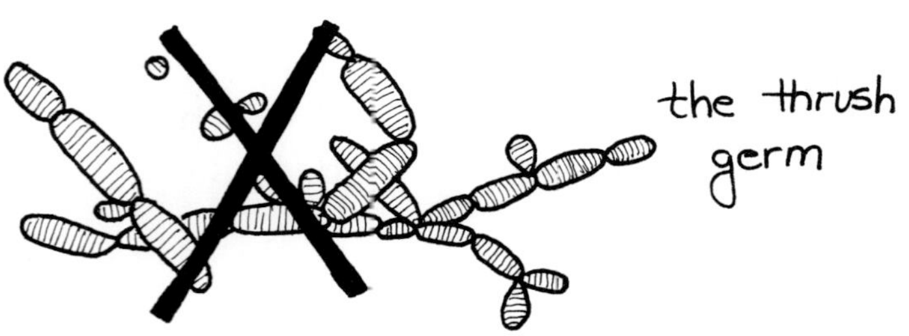

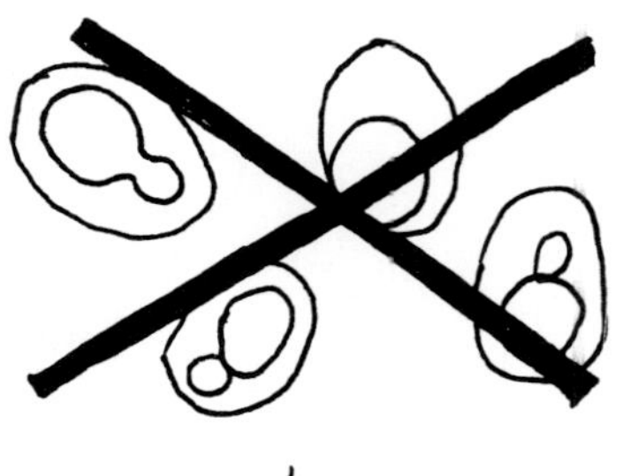

SCH 39304

has no other name yet.

It is an antifungal medicine

that is being *tested* to treat

brain infections caused by cryptococcus

in people with HIV.

It is given as a pill

and can be taken for a long time.

No one really knows yet what its side effects will be,

but scientists think side effects that SCH 39304 might cause are:

1. headaches
2. nausea
3. diarrhea

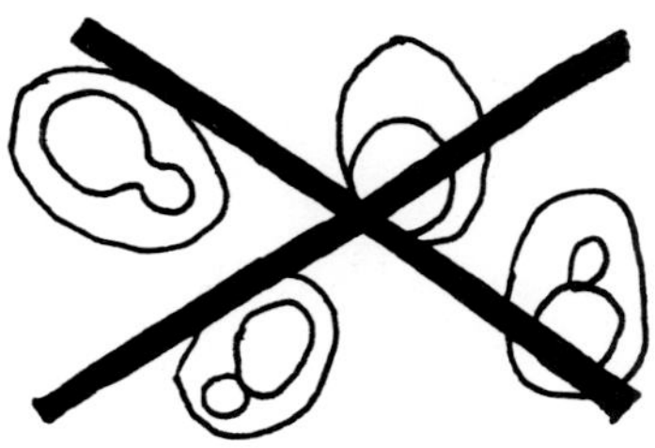

cryptococcus

Clindamycin

has many other names.

It is an antibiotic used to treat very serious infections

caused by bacteria in adults and children—

and it is being *tested* to treat PCP and toxoplasmosis

in people with HIV.

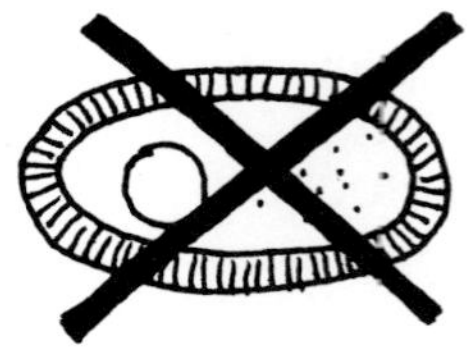

It comes as a pill, a liquid, IV or IM.

The liquid should *not* be kept in the refrigerator.

It is given three or four times a day

for several days.

P. carinii

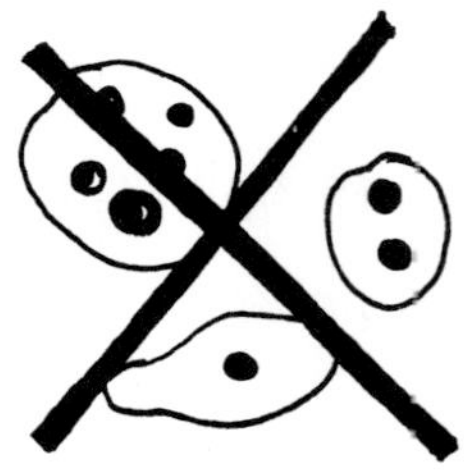

Side effects that clindamycin can cause are:

1. severe diarrhea
   (call your doctor if this happens)
2. nausea and vomiting
3. rash
4. severe allergic reaction
   in people allergic to lincomycin

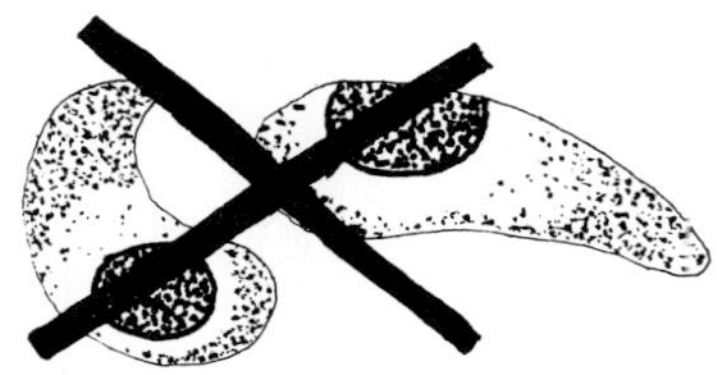

the toxoplasmosis germ

Other medicines that may not get along with clindamycin are:

erythromycin, ampicillin, phenytoin,

barbiturates, and aminophylline.

A medicine that can help clindamycin work better

is primaquine (a drug used to treat malaria).

They are sometimes used together

to treat people with PCP.

Dapsone

has many other names.

It is an antibiotic used to treat leprosy

and is now being *tested* to prevent and treat PCP

in people with HIV.

It comes as a pill

and is taken once or twice a day for a long time.

Side effects that dapsone can cause are:

1. rashes
2. itching
3. anemia
4. severe skin reactions

   (call your doctor if this happens to you)

Other medicines that may not get along with dapsone are:

pyrimethamine or any medicine that causes

the bone marrow to slow down its making of blood cells

such as AZT.

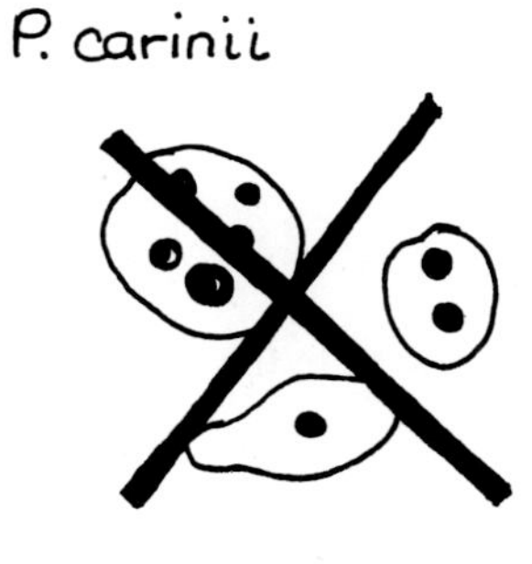

Fansidar

is a brand name for a combination of two medicines:

pyrimethamine and sulfadoxine.

Pyrimethamine is an antiprotozoal medicine

that is used to treat malaria and toxoplasmosis.

Sulfadoxine is an antibiotic

that is used to treat malaria.

The combination of the two, or Fansidar,

is being *tested* to prevent or treat PCP

in people with HIV.

It comes as a pill

and can be taken for a long time.

Fansidar should not be taken

by people who are allergic to sulfa medications.

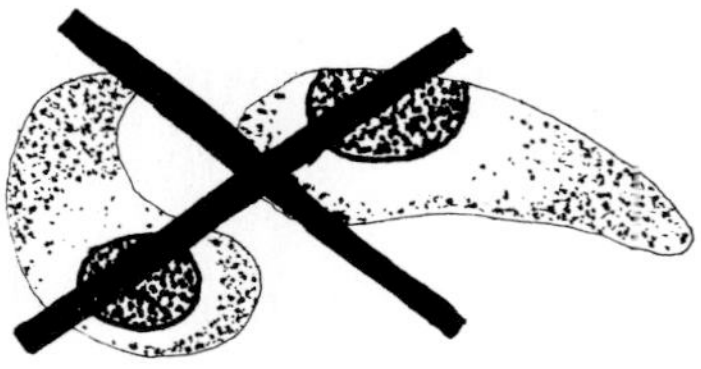

the toxoplasmosis germ

Side effects that Fansidar can cause are:

1. severe skin rash

   (call your doctor if this happens)

2. low blood counts
3. headache
4. stomachache
5. a mixed up feeling
6. fever and chills

P. carinii

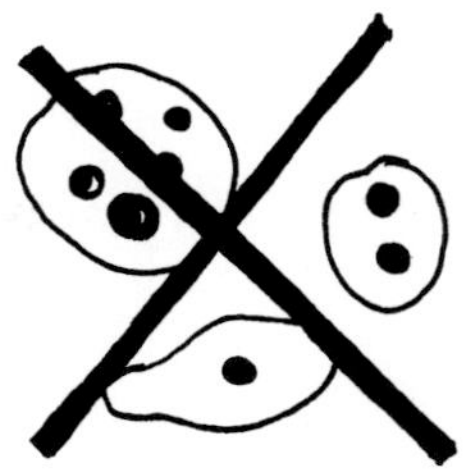

A medicine that should not be taken with Fansidar

is TMP/SMX.

A medicine that can reverse some side effects of Fansidar

is leukovorin.

DFMO

is also called eflornithine.

It is an antiprotozoal medicine

that is sometimes used

to treat HIV-infected people with PCP

who have not gotten better on other PCP medicines.

It comes as an IV or a pill

and can be given for a long time.

Side effects that DFMO can cause are:

1. slowing down of bone marrow in making blood cells
2. diarrhea
3. trouble hearing
4. seizures
5. rash

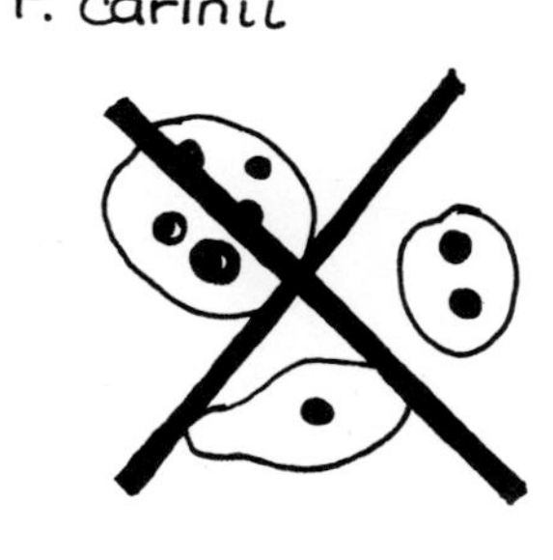

566C80

has no other name yet.

It is an antiprotozoal medicine

that is being *tested* to treat PCP

in people with HIV.

It is also being tested to treat toxoplasmosis.

It comes as a pill.

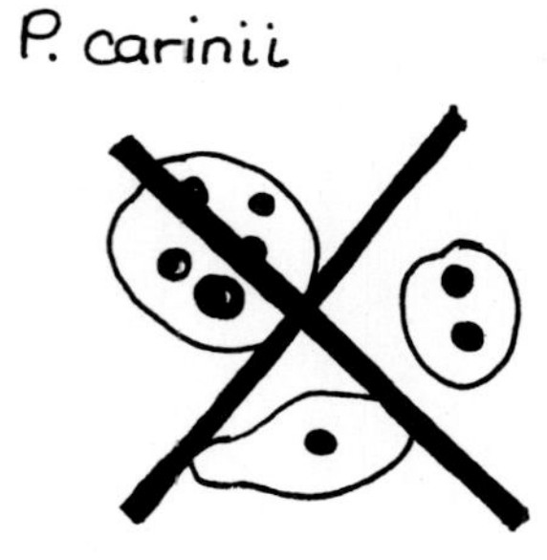

Pentamidine

is also called Pentam 300 and Lomidine.

It is an antiprotozoal medicine

that has been used for a long time

to treat PCP in children and adults—

including children and adults with HIV.

It is given IV or IM to treat PCP.

It also comes as an aerosol—

which is kind of like a mist that you breathe.

The aerosol kind of pentamidine is being used

to prevent PCP in people with HIV.

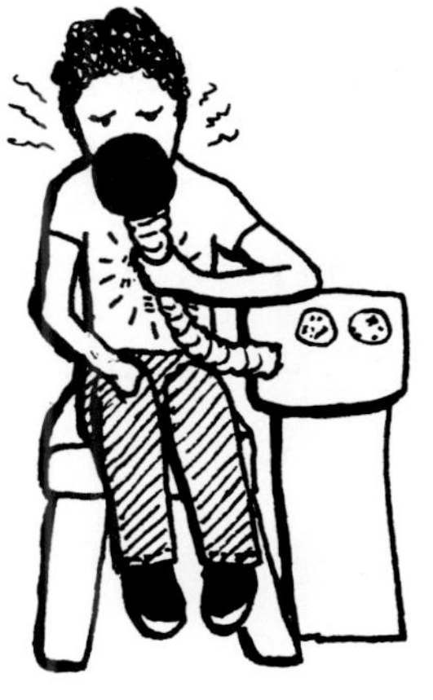

While the aerosol kind of pentamidine has few side effects,

pentamidine can have many side effects when given IV or IM.

Side effects that IV or IM pentamidine can cause are:

1. kidney problems
2. low blood counts
   (especially white cells and platelets)
3. low blood pressure (hypotension)
4. low blood sugar (hypoglycemia)
5. very fast heart rate
6. nervousness, dizziness or sleepiness
7. pain or swelling where the medicine was put in

Many medicines can make the side effects

of IV or IM pentamidine worse,

so always check with your doctor

before taking any new medicine

if you are getting IV or IM pentamidine.

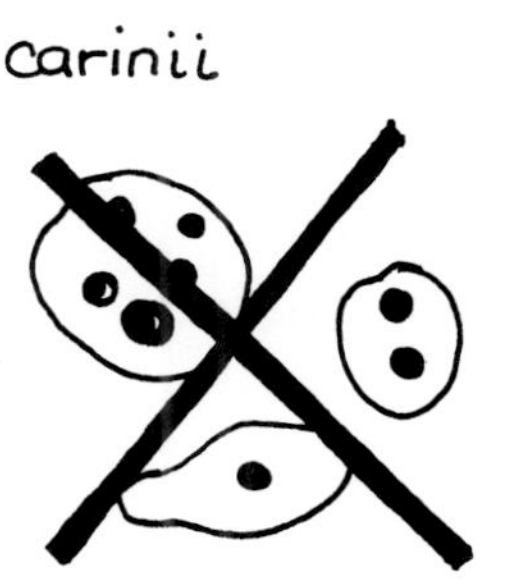

TMP-SMX

is also called trimethoprim-sulfamethoxazole.

It also has many other names, like Septra and Bactrim.

It is an antibiotic that is used to treat many infections

caused by bacteria in children and adults.

It is being used to both treat and prevent PCP

and to treat isosporiasis

in people with HIV.

It comes as a pill or a liquid.

The liquid does not need to be kept in the refrigerator,

but some kids like it better cold.

It's taken twice a day for a few weeks

or for a long time.

It is not given to babies younger than 2 months old.

P. carinii

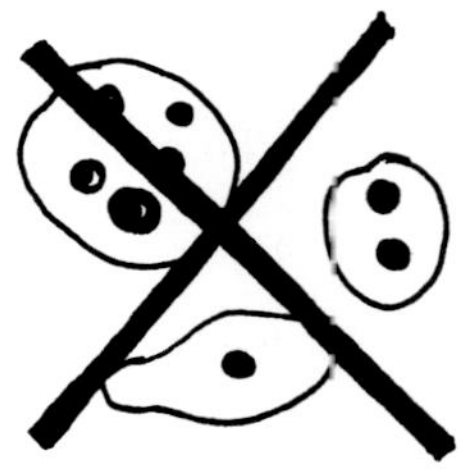

While many grownups have side effects from TMP-SMX,

most children don't

unless they are allergic to sulfa medications—

and then they shouldn't take it.

Side effects that TMP-SMX can cause are:

1. rash
2. fever
3. low white cell count

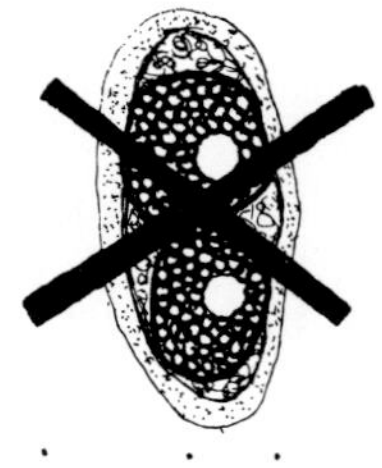

the isosporiasis germ

A medicine that may not get along with TMP-SMX is

phenytoin, a medicine used to prevent seizures.

Trimetrexate

has no other name yet.

It is being *tested* to treat many kinds of cancer

in both adults and children.

It is also being *tested* to treat PCP

in people with HIV.

It is given IV.

Side effects that trimetrexate can cause are:

1. rash
2. low blood counts

   (especially white cells and platelets)
3. stomachache
4. fever

In both people with cancer and people with HIV and PCP,

trimetrexate is used with another medicine

called leukovorin calcium

(which has many other names).

Leukovorin calcium protects people getting trimetrexate

from getting into too much trouble

because of low blood counts.

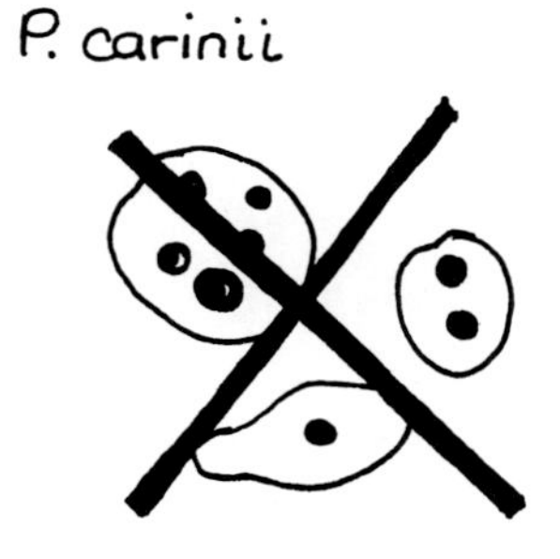

Spiramycin

has many other names.

It is an antibiotic

that is used to treat infections caused by bacteria.

It is sometimes used to treat cryptosporidiosis

in people with HIV.

It comes as a pill, IV, or SC (Sub-Q).

It is given for different lengths of time

depending on how you react to it.

Side effects that spiramycin can cause are:

1. fever
2. yellow skin or eyes

   (call your doctor if you get this)

Spiramycin cannot be given with ergotamine,

a medicine used to treat migraine headaches.

If you are taking bronchodilators,

such as theophylline,

or a heart medicine called digitalis,

spiramycin can make their side effects worse.

Your doctor will have to watch you carefully.

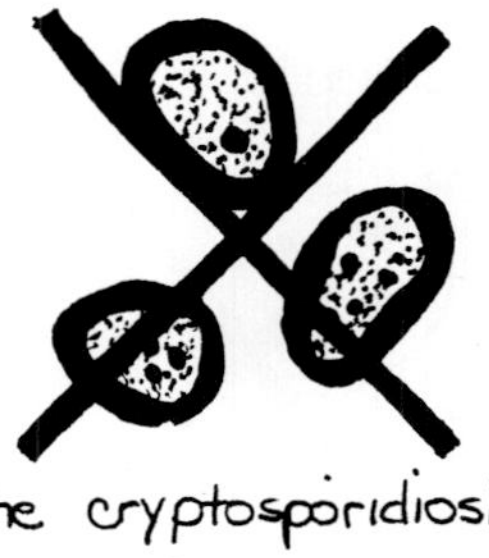

the cryptosporidiosis germ

Diclazuril

is also called Clinacox.

It is an antiprotozoal medicine

that is used to treat cryptosporidiosis infections

in animals.

It is being *tested* to treat cryptosporidiosis

in people with HIV.

It comes as a pill.

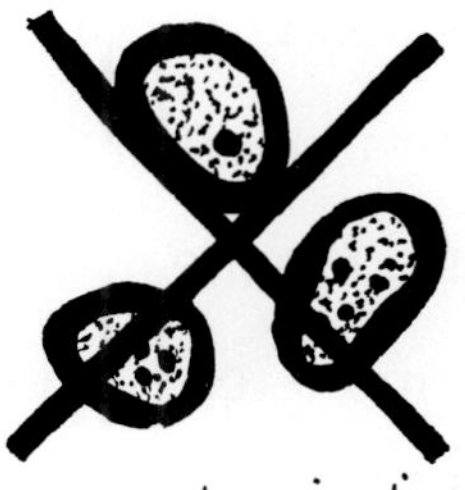

New Anti-Infectives

2. Other Medicines

Erythropoietin

is also called Eprex or EPO.

It is a hormone our livers and kidneys make

that tells our bone marrow

to make more red blood cells.

It is made by bacteria

that have had the part of our DNA plan

that causes our bodies to make erythropoietin

put into their own DNA plans

by something called genetic engineering.

(Genetic engineering is nothing more

than people doing the same thing

viruses have been doing forever.)

It is used to treat anemia in many people,

including people with HIV.

It is given IV or SC (Sub-Q).

(Many kids think the SC shots hurt

and would rather get their Eprex IV.)

The only side effect erythropoietin has ever caused

is a mild skin rash.

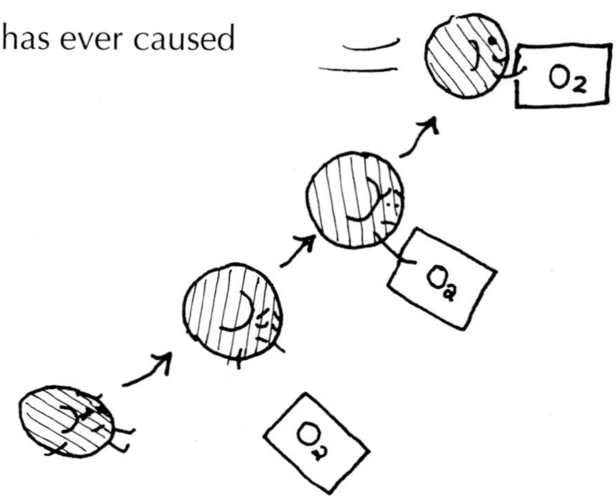

Prednisone

is also called PRED.

It is used to treat many different diseases

where a whole bunch of lymphocytes get together in a place

where there shouldn't be any, or only a few,

such as some kinds of arthritis.

It is sometimes used to treat LIP,

because in LIP the lungs fill up with lymphocytes

and that makes it hard to breathe.

It comes as a pill.

It is usually taken for many days

and then you may have to *taper,* or slowly decrease,

the amount of PRED you take

until you don't take it for a while.

Tapering is easy—it's done by twos:

every two days, you divide the dose in half.

(You may want to use a calendar to keep track of this.)

Side effects that PRED can cause are:

1. big appetite and weight gain
2. tummy aches
3. not feeling sick

   even though you have an infection
4. mood changes (feeling too happy or too cranky)
5. fragile bones, if you take PRED a long time
6. high blood pressure (hypertension)
7. high blood sugar (hyperglycemia)

New Medicines

3. Blood Transfusions

Blood transfusions are often important
for people with HIV.
So you should know
something about them.

To begin with,
blood that is used for transfusions
is given by healthy people who are called donors.
A donor usually gives a pint of blood at one time
(that's about two measuring cups full).
The blood can be used right away,
or, if it is kept cold,
the blood can be used up to three weeks
after it is donated.
The blood is stored in a special place
called a blood bank.

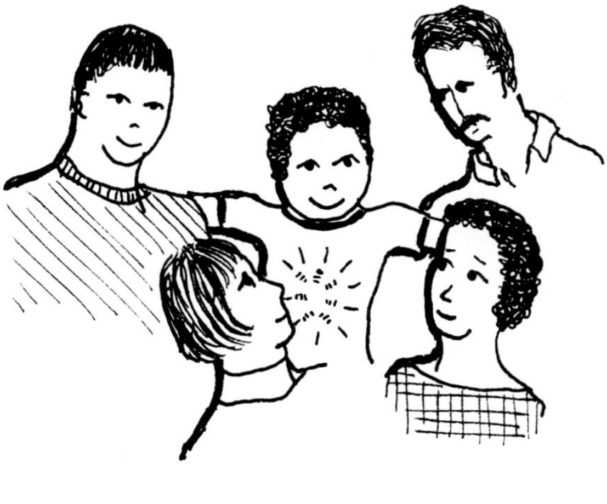

Blood, as you know,
is made up of many parts.
Whole blood, which contains all the different parts,
is usually not used for transfusion
except for people who have lost a lot of blood.
Those people need *all* the different things
in the donor's blood.
But most people, whether or not they have HIV,
don't need whole blood.
Usually, only one part of their blood is missing—
like RBCs are missing in anemia
or platelets are missing in thrombocytopenia.
It makes a lot of sense
to separate all the different things in blood.
That way blood from one donor
can help more than one other person.
The red cells can be given to someone with anemia.
The platelets can be given to someone else
who has thrombocytopenia.
It makes a lot of sense
and it's exactly what doctors do.
Usually, your transfusion will have only the part of blood
that *you* need.

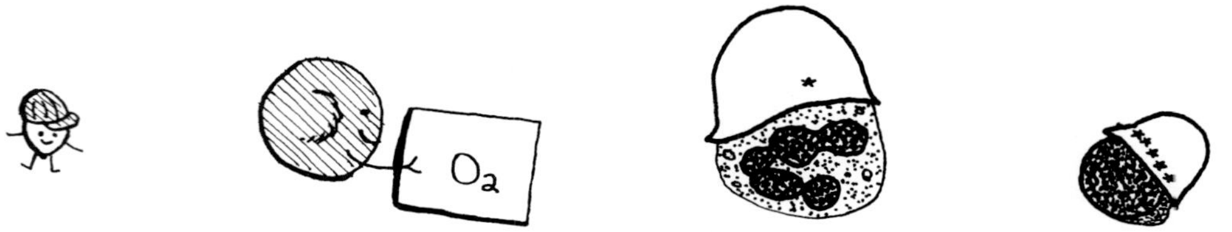

What happens during a blood transfusion
is the same whether you're getting whole blood
or just one part (component).
A bottle or plastic bag
that contains blood chosen especially for you
is hung upside down at the top of a tall pole.
A long skinny tube is connected
to the blood at one end
and to you at the other.
Since blood has to go into your veins
if it's going to do any good,
you will have to have an IV needle in one of your veins
or, if you have one,
your central line can be used.
The blood is allowed to flow into your body slowly.
That way, if any problem starts,
the transfusion can be stopped
before you get very much of the donor blood.
Even though problems don't happen very often,
no one wants to take any chances with you.
If you are going to have a blood transfusion,
you might want to bring a book to look at
while the blood drips in,
just as you do if you get IVIG.

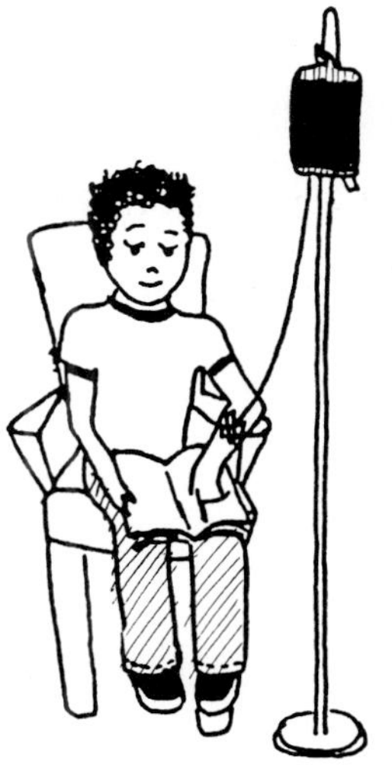

Blood transfusions,
like almost everything else in medicine,
can cause problems of their own.
For this reason, they're never used
unless they are really needed.
Blood transfusions can cause two main kinds of problems.
One is that if the donor had a disease,
such as hepatitis (a liver disease caused by a virus)
or HIV (which you already know *a lot* about),
the germs that caused the disease may still be in the blood.
So, you could get the disease.
No one wants this to happen.
Donors are chosen who appear to be healthy,
but sometimes a donor has a disease
and doesn't know it.
And the doctor doesn't know it.
So, all donated blood is tested
to see if it has these germs in it.
But, no matter how careful everyone is,
there is always a very small risk
of spreading a disease
by transfusing blood.
But, it almost never happens anymore.

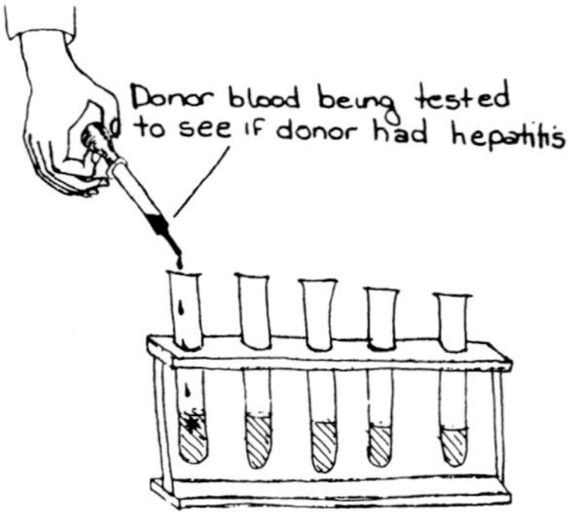

The second type of problem happens
when your own immune system
decides that the cells in the transfused blood
are enemies
and tries to destroy them.
This is called a transfusion reaction.
If you think about it,
this kind of problem makes a lot of sense.
The cells in the blood transfusion
are someone else's blood cells,
not yours.
It is your immune system's job
to find and destroy all strange cells.
So, if your immune system
tries to destroy transfused blood cells,
it's just doing what it's supposed to do—
and you can't really blame it.

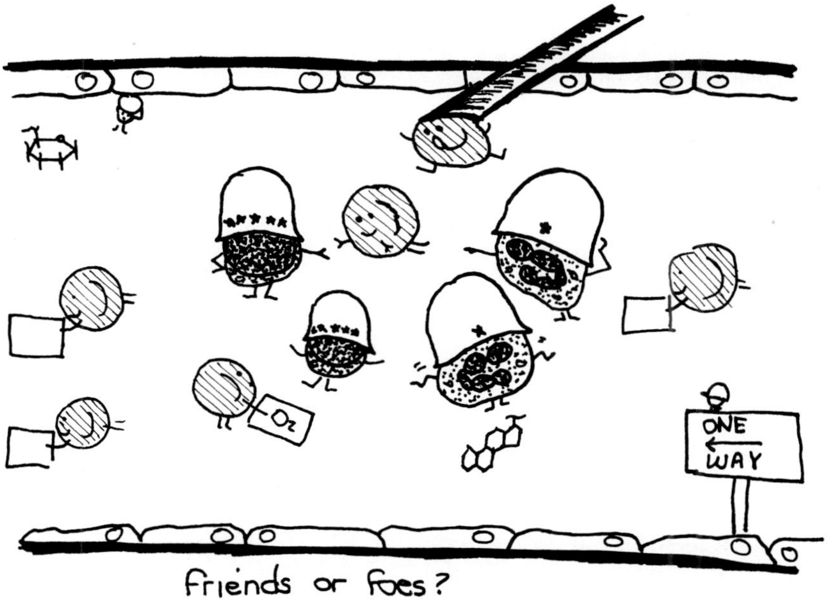

friends or foes?

However, you are having a blood transfusion
because you need those blood cells.
They can't help you if they're destroyed.
So, doctors have studied all the cells in blood
and figured out what most of their antigens are.
Before you get a blood transfusion,
your doctors will find out which antigens you have
on your own blood cells.
This is your blood type (for RBCs)
and tissue type (for WBCs and platelets).
Then, they will find out which antigens
are on the donor's blood cells.
This is the donor's blood type (for RBCs)
and tissue type (for WBCs and platelets).
The donor blood chosen for you
will have the same blood or tissue type that you do.
This means that the blood cells that will be given to you
will have the same antigens on them
as your own blood cells do.
This way, your immune system
will think the donor cells are friends, not enemies,
and leave them alone so they can help you.

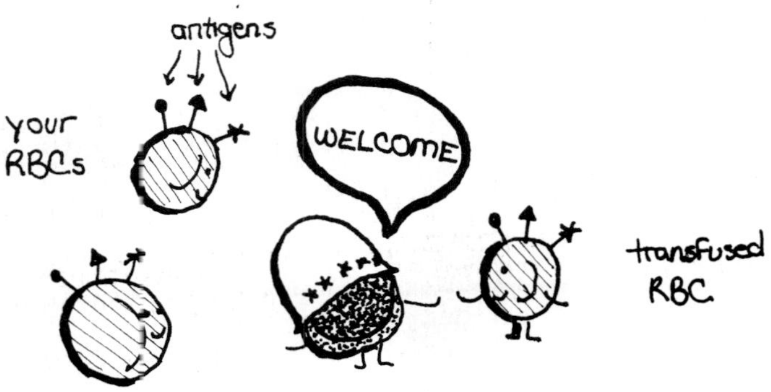

Even though doctors have gotten really good
at matching blood and tissue types of donors
with the blood and tissue types
of the people who get the donor's blood,
it's not yet perfect.
Doctors haven't yet figured out every single antigen
on every single blood cell.
So, transfusion reactions can still happen.

Symptoms of a transfusion reaction are:

1. nausea and vomiting
2. fever
3. skin rash and itching
4. a feeling that someone is sitting on your chest
5. yellow skin or eyes
6. pain in your lower back

Transfusion reactions
hardly ever happen—
but if you have any of these feelings
while getting a blood transfusion,
tell your doctor right away.

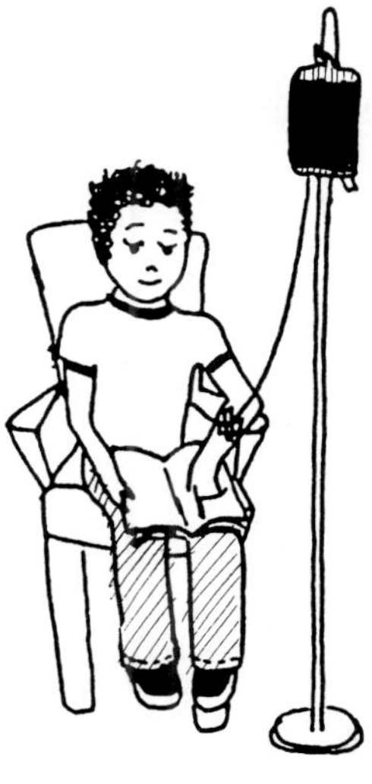

It's hard for anyone to know
whether you will ever need a blood transfusion at all,
or if you'll need just a few,
or if you'll need to have a lot of them.
Even so, now you and your family know
how important it is to have blood waiting for you
in the blood bank in case you need it.
Blood for transfusions can only come from people—
people who care about other people.
If it's possible, you might want to ask
your relatives or family friends
to donate their blood to the blood bank.
In a way, it will replace the blood given to *you.*
The people who care about you
often feel frustrated and helpless.
They sometimes think there's nothing they can do to help.
Tell them that donating blood to the blood bank
is one way they can help.
Tell them that they can't get HIV
by *donating* blood.
(Of course, if they also have HIV,
they should not donate blood.
That would not help you,
and it could make someone else sick.
But there are, after all, many ways
that people who love one another can help
besides blood transfusions.)

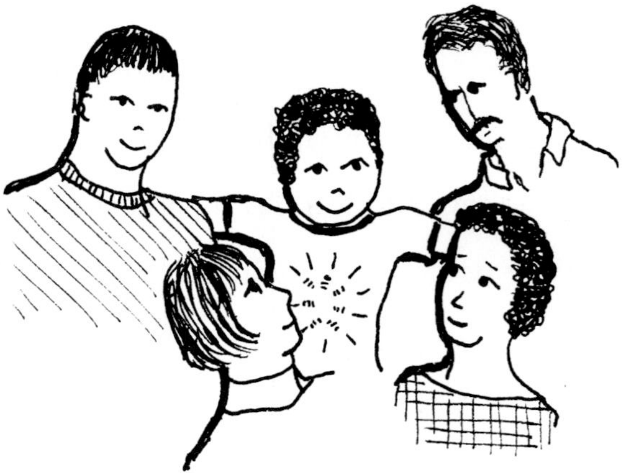

4. *Central Lines*

Many of the medicines you need
to treat HIV or its complications
need to be given as shots into a vein (IV).
So do blood transfusions.
Also, if you get bad diarrhea
or just can't eat anything,
you may need to be given liquid IV "food"
(which is called parenteral nutrition
or hyperalimentation).
Many of the blood tests you will need to have
also mean taking blood out of a vein.
After a while, people with HIV
can start feeling like pin cushions.
So, doctors figured out a way to do all this
that lets people feel like people,
not like pin cushions.
They way they do this
is by using something called
a central line
or indwelling venous catheter.

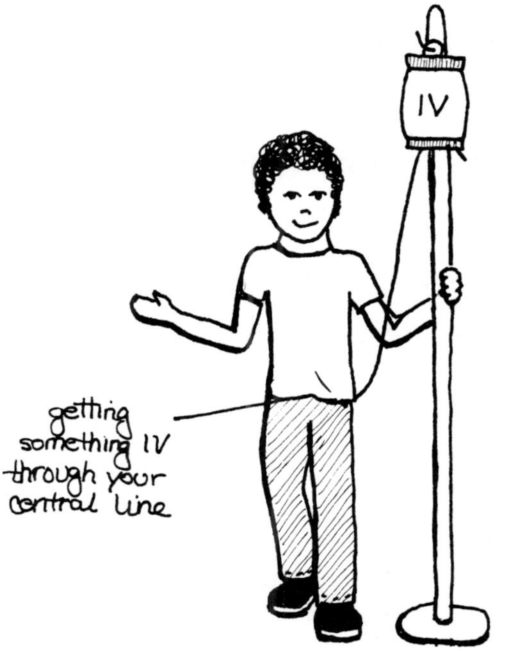

A catheter is a soft plastic tube.
It's hollow like a straw
but also bendy like half-way cooked spaghetti.
Catheters are used for lots of things,
like getting urine out of your bladder
if it forgets to push it out itself.
An IV is actually a little catheter
than can only be in place for a few days.
A central line is a longer catheter.
It is put into one of the big veins in your chest
and can stay there for a very long time.
Actually, only one end of the catheter
is in a big vein.
The other end either comes a little way out
of the skin on your chest,
or just ends at your chest
or ends just under the skin of your chest.
This is the only part that you can see,
and it is the part that is used
to give you all the things you need
that must be given into a vein.
The catheter, or central line,
takes the place of lots of shots.
These catheters have lots of names.
Common ones are: Broviac, Hickman and Porta-Cath.

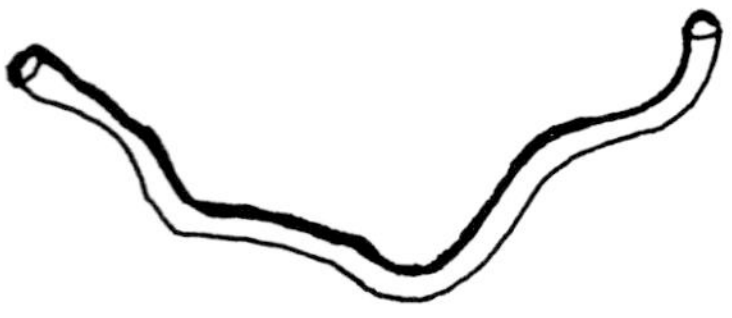

The central line is put into place

by a surgeon.

Surgeons, you remember, are doctors who do operations.

It takes an operation to put in a central line.

Because operations can be painful,

the first thing that will happen to you

(once you and everyone else are in the funny blue clothes)

is that you will be given something so you don't feel pain.

You might be given a numbing medicine

to make the nerves where the doctor will work

fall sound asleep, as in a bone marrow test.

Or you might be given a medicine that makes

you fall asleep, as in an open lung biopsy.

The kind of anesthesia, or "no pain" medicine

that you will get

will depend on what your doctors think is best for you.

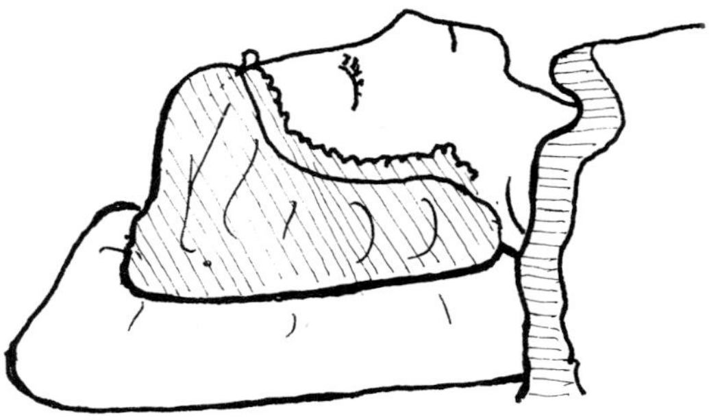

Once you are feeling no pain,
the surgeon will make two small cuts in your skin.
One is usually near your right shoulder
over the spot where your catheter will go into your vein.
The other is usually near the middle of your chest,
where the catheter will either end
or come out of your body.
Through these two small openings,
the surgeon will put the catheter in place.
Once it's there, the surgeon has to make sure
it stays where it's supposed to.
Surgeons do that by stitching, which is kind of like sewing,
the catheter to the vein (where it goes in)
and to your skin (if you have the kind that comes out)
or to the muscles under your skin (if you have a Porta-Cath).
The only stitches you will see
will be the ones on your skin.

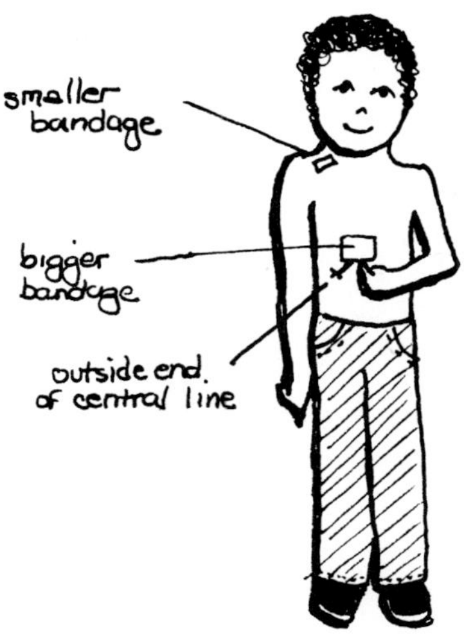

When the operation is over,
you will have two bandages.
There will be a small one near your right shoulder
and a bigger one on your chest
over the spot where the catheter ends.
The skin under these bandages
may be kind of sore for a few days,
the way the skin near any cut is sore at first.
The small cut near your shoulder will heal fast.
So will the skin over your Porta-Cath, if you have one.
If you have a catheter that comes out,
it can take many weeks to heal completely,
but most of that time it won't hurt.
It takes a long time because the inside of your skin
has to kind of glue itself to the catheter
so that the central line won't slide out
after the stitches holding it in are removed.
Whatever kind of catheter you have,
you won't have to wait until the stitches come out
to use it.
It will be ready to use right away!

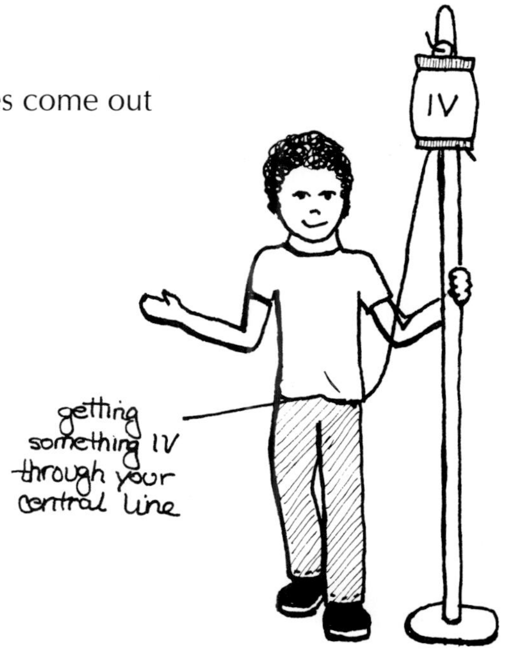

The first thing you'll notice about having a central line
is that your arms are free again,
even when you're getting something IV.
The second thing you'll notice
is that you won't be getting very many shots anymore
(if you have the kind that ends at your skin)
or that your shots don't hurt as much
(if you have the kind that ends just under your skin).
That's because all the stuff you used to get IV
can now be given using your central line.
And, blood can be taken out of it
when you need a blood test.
When you go home with your central line,
you'll be able to do everything you did before,
except for rough sports like football or wrestling.
But gentler sports are safe.
Your catheter will be hidden under your clothes or your skin
so no one will even know you have it
unless you want to show it to them.

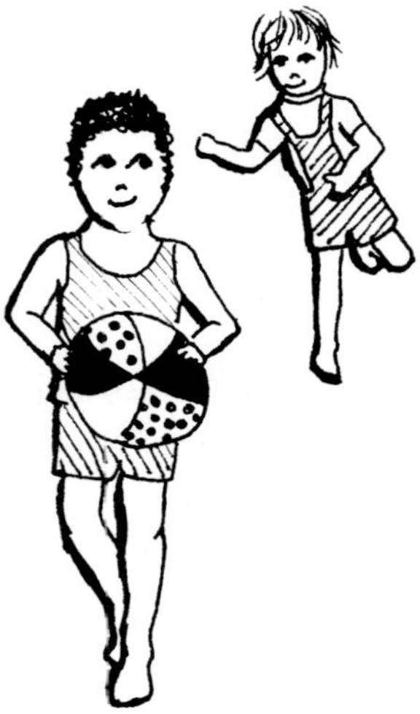

If your central line ends at or comes out of your skin,
it will need to be taken care of every day
so that it can stay in place for a long time,
and so that it doesn't get infected.

In the hospital, your nurses will do your catheter care.
At home, you and your parents or caretakers
will need to do it.
There are two goals in catheter care.
One is keeping it clean,
which is done by changing the bandage often.
The other is keeping it open,
which is done by putting a small amount
of a medicine called heparin
into the catheter.
Heparin is a medicine that stops blood from clumping,
which could plug up your central line.
Central line, or catheter, care
is not hard to do.
Your nurses will teach you all how to do it
until you are as good at it as they are.
If you have a Porta-Cath,
you won't have to do the keeping clean part—
but you will still have to do the keeping open part.

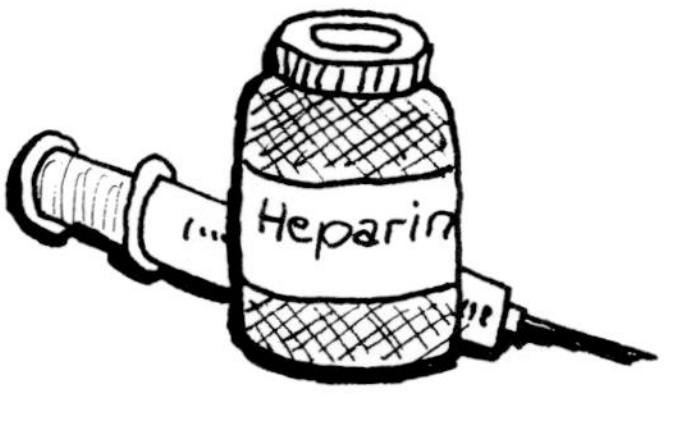

5. Oxygen

Oxygen is the stuff in the air we breathe
that our cells need to use to get energy out of food
(see page 13).
Sometimes when people's lungs aren't working well,
as in PCP, LIP, and other problems,
they need to breathe in more oxygen
than other people do.
Since there is only a certain amount of oxygen in air,
the way people who need more oxygen get it
is from oxygen tanks.
Oxygen tanks are kind of like scuba diving tanks.
They can be big or little.
Some kinds can be wheeled around
so you can take your oxygen with you.
There is a tube from the tank that goes to your nose
where it divides into two little tubes
that fit inside the holes in your nose.
These tubes are held in place by an elastic band
that goes around your head.

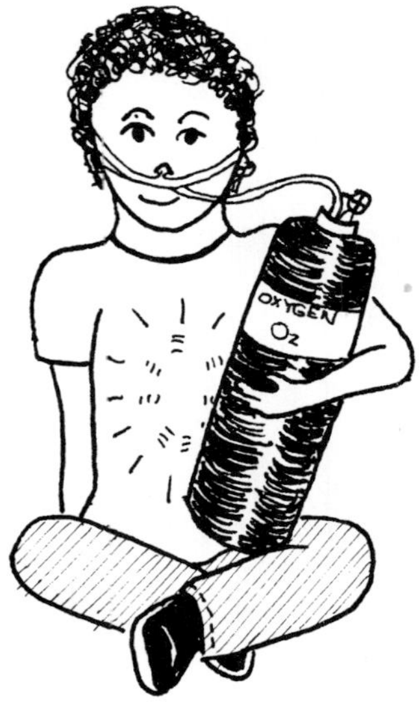

Not all children with HIV need to use oxygen,
so you may not.
But, if you do, you'll find it helps you feel
more alert and have more energy.
You'll also find that it can be kind of a pain
to cart your oxygen around with you all the time,
but if it helps you feel better,
it's worth the trouble.
Most people don't have to use the oxygen
every single minute of every day.
And as your lung condition improves,
you won't need to use it as much either.
Oxygen doesn't have any side effects,
but it can cause other problems.
Sometimes other kids might tease you about the tank.
That can make you feel mad or bad,
but you can tell them and yourself
that it's more important to *feel* good
than it is to *look* good.
Sometimes other kids get jealous
because you have a tank and they don't.
It might make you and them feel better about this
if you let them help you wheel it around sometimes.

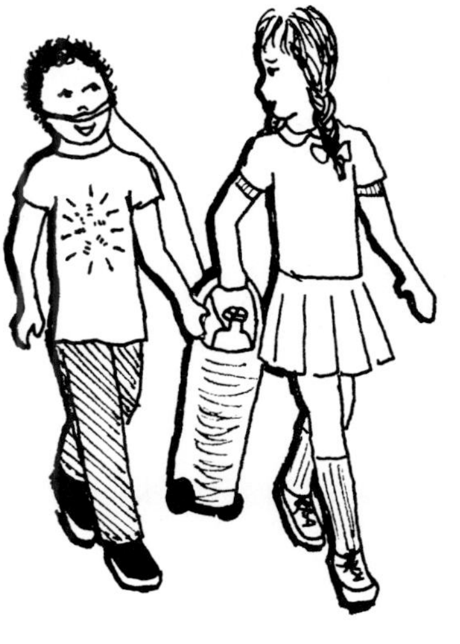

6. Pain Management

Pain hurts.

It hurts to have it.

It hurts to think about it.

It even can hurt to talk or read about it.

But thinking, talking, and reading about pain

is important

if you don't want to have to feel it.

Some of the complications of HIV are painful.

Some of the things doctors do

to diagnose and treat these complications

are also painful.

Sometimes, pain lasts only a few days;

other times it can last for weeks.

Some pains hurt all the time;

others come and go.

Some hurt just a little;

others hurt a lot.

If you are having pain,

don't keep it a secret—*tell* someone,

your family, your doctor, your nurses.

Much can and should be done

to make you more comfortable—

no matter what kind of pain you are having.

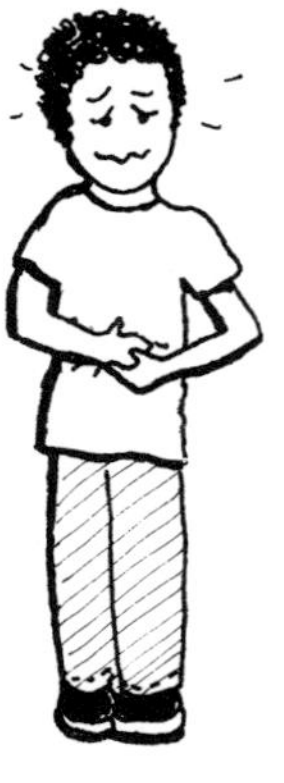

Pain medicines are one thing
that can help you feel better.
There are three main kinds of pain medicines.

The first is over-the-counter (O.T.C.) pain medicines.
These are the ones you don't need a doctor's prescription for.
Aspirin, acetaminophen and ibuprofen
are all O.T.C. pain medicines.
All are excellent for most kinds of pain.
All come as liquids, as pills you can chew,
or as pills you can swallow, if you know how.
Some also come as suppositories (see page 133).
These are very powerful medicines,
even though you don't need a prescription to buy them.
You should ask your doctor which one to use,
because it will depend on what other medicines you are taking
and what other problems you are having besides pain.

The second is prescription, non-narcotic pain medicines.
Most of these are stronger forms of ibuprofen.
Another one is naproxen.
They are given as liquids or pills.

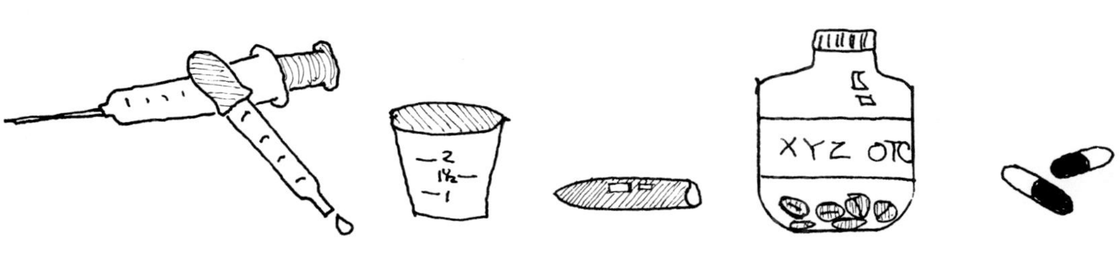

The third is prescription, narcotic pain medicines.
These are the strongest of them all.
Codeine, morphine, Demerol and methadone
are examples of prescription, narcotic medicines.
They can be given as liquids, pills, suppositories,
shots into a muscle (IM) or IV.
Narcotics have kind of a bad rap.
This isn't because they are bad medicines.
It is because some people use them
for the wrong reasons.
These people are called "drug abusers."
Some drug abusers become "drug addicts,"
which means, they can't stop abusing narcotics.
But people who take prescription narcotics
that their doctors give them to control pain
are not drug abusers or drug addicts.
They are just patients,
people who are using narcotics
the way they were meant to be used.

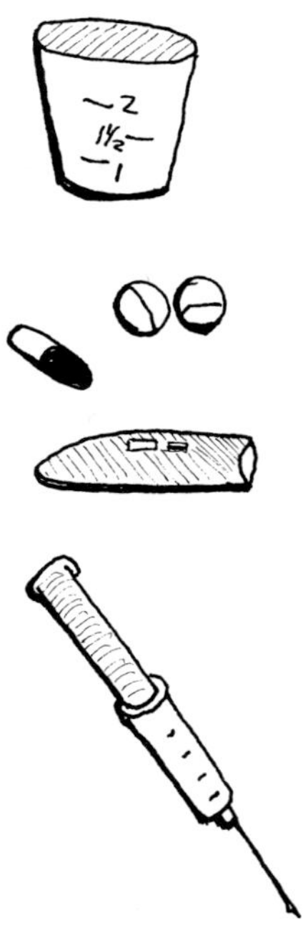

All pain medications should be taken
in the amount the doctor tells you to take it,
at the times your doctor tells you to take it,
and for as long as your doctor tells you to take it.

All pain medicines should be given
in the way that will be the least painful to you.

All pain medicines should be taken often enough
that you don't start hurting again.

You need to talk with your doctor
and the rest of your treatment team
about all of these things.

Also, your pain medicines are meant for you
and no one else.
Other people in your family
should not take your medicines
(whether they're pain medicines or other kinds).
And all your medicines should be kept in a safe place,
with "childproof" caps on them.

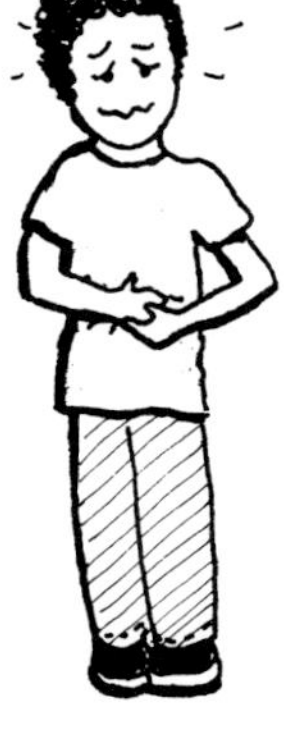

Besides pain medicines,
there are other things your family can do
to help you feel better if you are hurting.
When people hurt,
their bodies and minds get all tense and nervous.
This can make the pain hurt even more.
Helping your body and mind relax
is one way your family can help ease your pain.

Mild heat is often helpful for pain.
A heating pad on a sore place
or a long, warm bath
can help your body relax.

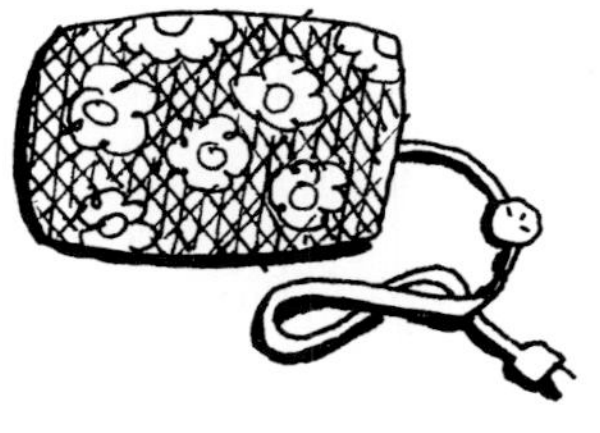

Gentle back rubs, neck rubs, and head rubs
can also help your body relax
and make you feel better.

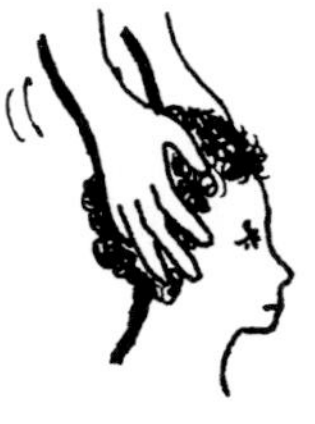

Just being held and quietly cuddled
can help a person feel safe and loved.
These are relieving feelings.
And while kisses probably
never really make a pain go away,
they always make the person with the pain
feel better.

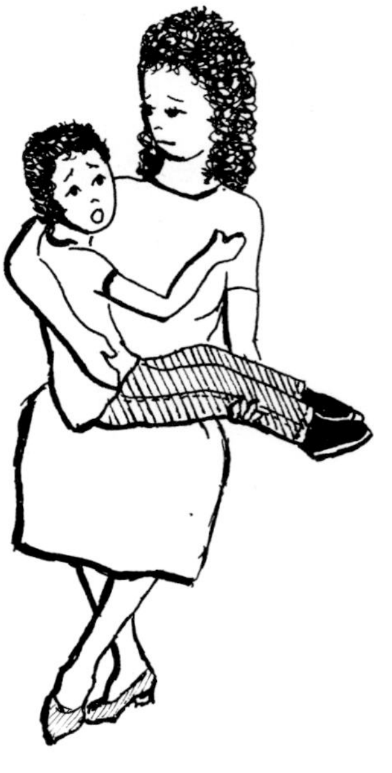

There are also things you can do yourself
to help your body hurt less.

One is to be sure to remember to breathe.
That may sound silly,
because who would ever forget to breathe?
But when people are in pain,
they often hold their breath a lot.
This can make the pain hurt more.
So just remembering to breathe,
slowly and evenly,
can help a lot.

Another is to let yourself cry,
if you feel like you need to.
Crying does two things.
One is that it makes you breathe.
The other is that, when you're finished,
your body will feel much more relaxed
than it did when you were trying not to cry.
Crying doesn't mean you're a baby or a wimp.
Crying is a way our bodies have
to get rid of the tension pain can cause.

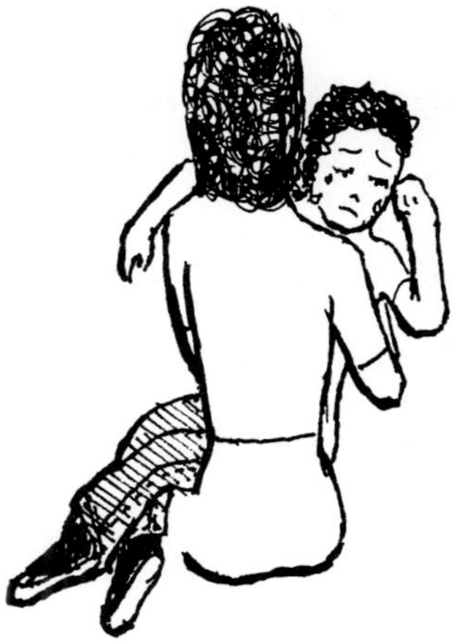

Another thing you can do

is to use your brain to help your pain go away.

Your brain is the part of you that thinks.

If all your brain is thinking about is how much you hurt,

you will feel worse.

You can help your brain think about other things.

You can get it so busy thinking about those other things

that it can forget to think about pain.

And if your brain isn't thinking about pain,

you won't be feeling pain.

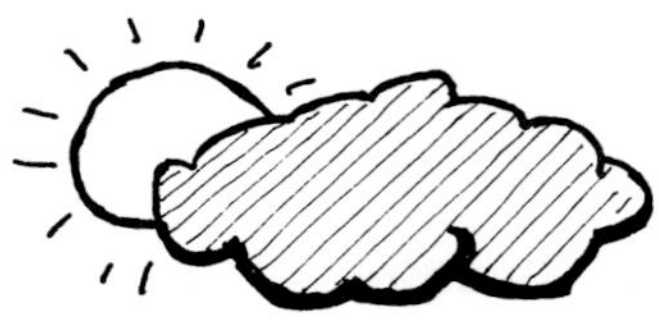

Think of something that is beautiful to you,

such as a big fluffy cloud floating in a blue, blue sky.

Then close your eyes and just watch what you have imagined.

Once you get good at that, you can do more.

Imagine that your pain is a fire—

and then imagine yourself blowing it out.

Or have your pain be laser beams

and imagine them flying out of your body

and going away into outer space.

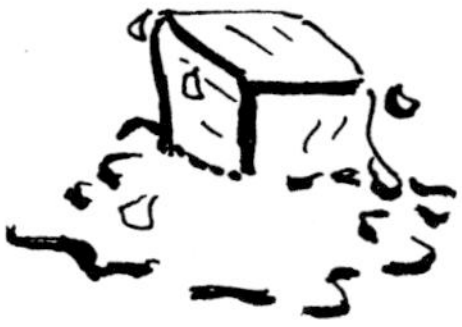

Your pain might be a ice cube—that melts.

Or a slinky that relaxes into a floppy string.

You can use these images—or make up your own.

It can be fun to do,

and even more important,

it really can help you feel better.

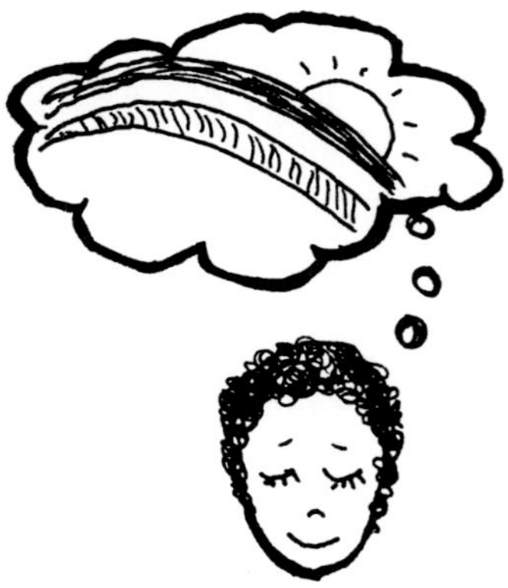

You can also use the power of your mind
to try to help your immune system get rid of HIV
and to try to help your medicines work better.
This book has told you
how your immune system works,
what HIV and other germs look like and do,
and how your medicines work.
You can imagine the cells of your immune system
eating up all the germs they find.
You can imagine your medicines
doing what they're supposed to do.
You can use the pictures from this book,
or make up your very own images.
For example, if you don't like soldiers,
you can imagine the cells of your immune system
being vacuum cleaners that vacuum up germs
and then imagine throwing them in the trash.

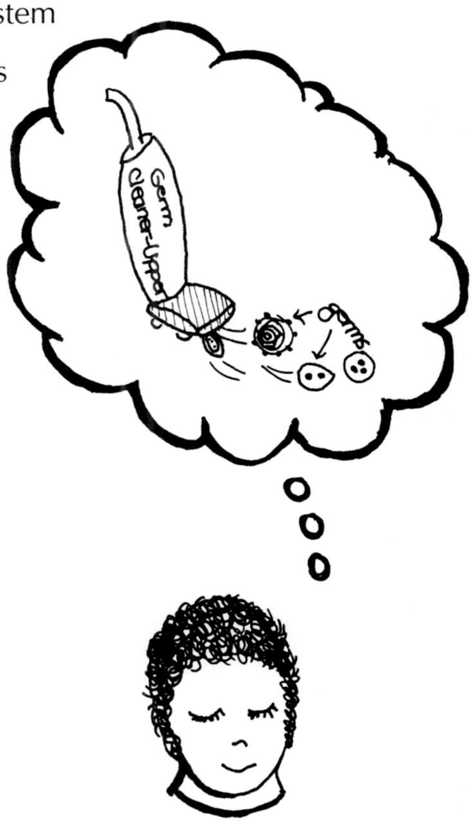

Will this help you get better?

No one can say for sure.

What is known is that it will help you *feel* better.

That's important.

You and your doctors are already

doing so many things to help you get better.

So, it's only fair

that you spend at least as much time

thinking about getting well

as you do thinking about being sick.

That is, when you aren't too busy

playing games, giggling with friends,

and doing all the other things

that make life so wonderful.

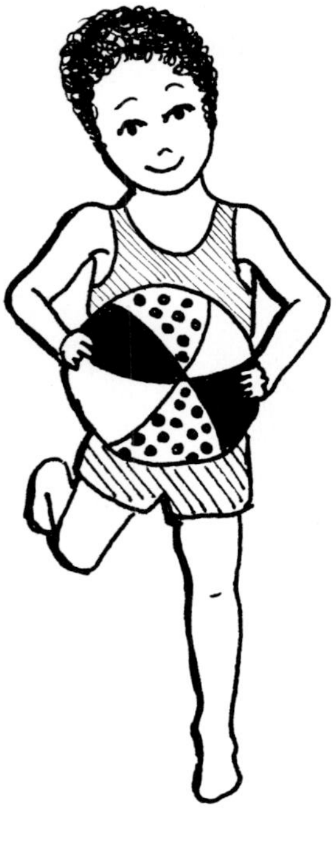

FURTHER READING

This is a list of books that should be available in your local bookstore or library. Some of them are specifically about HIV and others are about related subjects. This is by no means a list of all the books ever written on these subjects, only those I have personally read and believe to be of potential interest to you and your family.

Books for Children (and Older People)

Allison, L: *Blood and Guts, A working Guide to Your Own Insides.* Boston, Little, Brown and Company, 1976.

Berenstain, S, and Berenstain, J: *The Berenstain Bears Go to the Doctor.* New York, Random House, 1981.

Berger, M: *Germs Make Me Sick!* New York, Harper and Row, 1985.

Bernstein, JE, and Gullo, SV: *When People Die.* New York, E.P. Dutton, 1977. For parents and children to read together.

Buscaglia, L: *The Fall of Freddie the Leaf.* Thorofare, New Jersey, Charles B. Slack, Inc., 1982. A simple story about life and death, for parents and children to read together.

Ciliotta, C, and Livingston, C: *Why Am I Going to the Hospital?* Secaucus, New Jersey, Lyle Stuart, Inc., 1981. A book written with wit and wisdom about how children feel about hospitals.

Elting, M: *The Macmillan Book of the Human Body.* New York, Macmillan Publishing Company, 1986. A beautifully illustrated anatomy book for kids.

Grollman, E: *Talking About Death.* Boston, Beacon Press, 1971. Rabbi Grollman's book is for children and parents to read together. (Another of his books, *Explaining Death to Children,* is just for adults.)

Harlow, R: *My Doctor.* New York, Macmillan Company, Inc., 1973. About what doctors do. For little kids.

Hauscherr, R: *Children and the AIDS Virus.* New York, Clarion Books, 1989. This is a wonderful educational book.

Jenness, A: *Families.* Boston, Houghton Mifflin Company, 1990. A book, with photographs, that celebrates many different kinds of families.

Kaufman, J: *How We Are Born, How We Grow, How Our Bodies Work, and How We Learn.* New York, Golden Press, 1975.

Kübler-Ross, E: *Remember the Secret.* Millbrae, California, Celestial Arts, 1982. A very spiritual (and nicely illustrated) story about two children who must face the reality of death.

LeShan, E: *What Makes Me Feel This Way? Growing Up with Human Emotions.* New York, Collier Books, 1972.

MacDonald, MR: *The Origin of Johnny.* New York, Alfred A. Knopf, 1975. About genes, heredity and DNA. For older kids and parents.

Mayer, M: *There Is a Nightmare in My Closet.* New York, Dial Books for Young Readers, 1968. A funny book about how a child learns to cope with his biggest fear.

Mayle, P: *Where Did I Come From?* Secaucus, New Jersey, Lyle Stuart, Inc., 1973. The facts of life, for children. Two other books in this series by the same author are *What's Happening to Me?,* about puberty, for older children; and *Will I Go to Heaven?* (New York, Corwin Books, 1976), about what death and heaven mean to different people. These are great books about often embarrassing subjects that both kids and adults will actually enjoy reading together.

Nilsson, L: *A Child Is Born.* New York, Dell Publishing Company, 1977. A beautifully photographed book about life before birth. I think this book is for everyone. You'll have to decide for you.

Schilling, S, and Swain, J: *My Name Is Jonathan (and I Have AIDS).* Denver, Prickly Pair Publishing & Consulting Company, 1989. Jonathan Swain tells about his life with AIDS.

Simon, N: *The Saddest Time.* Niles, Illinois, Albert Whitman & Company, 1986. Stories about children who lose people they know and love to death, and how they feel about and cope with their losses.

Stein, SB: *About Dying.* New York, Walker & Company, 1974. For children and parents to read together, with photographs.

Tasker, M: *Jimmy and the Eggs Virus.* This is one of the first books written for children with HIV. You can get a copy by writing to: C.H.A.P., Children's Hospital of New Jersey, United Hospitals Medical Center, 15 South 9th Street, Newark, NJ 07107; or by calling: (201) 268-8273.

Books for Teenagers (and Older People)

Blake, J: *Risky Times: How to Be AIDS-Smart and Stay Healthy.* New York, Workman Publishing, 1990. A guide for teenagers.

de Sainte Phalle, N: *AIDS, You Can't Catch It Holding Hands.* San Francisco and Santa Monica, California, The Lapis Press, 1987. An informational book about HIV transmission. While simply written, its lively illustrations sometimes make it hard to read.

Glasser, RJ: *The Body Is the Hero.* New York, Random House, 1976. A super book about immunology that reads like a detective story.

Hein, K, DiGeronimo, T, and the Editors of Consumers Report Books: *AIDS: Trading Fears for Facts, A Guide for Teens.* Mount Vernon, New York, Consumer's Union, 1989.

Hoffman, A: *At Risk.* New York, G.P. Putnam's Sons, 1988. A novel about a little girl with HIV.

Thomas, L: *The Lives of a Cell: Notes of a Biology Watcher.* New York, Bantam Books, Inc., 1974. A delightful book about life and living things, by a man who is one of our most respected scientists and observers of life's processes.

Books just for Adults

Anderson, P: *Children's Hospital.* New York, Harper and Row, 1985. A nurse writes of her experiences working with a variety of very sick children and their families.

Callen, M: *Surviving and Thriving with AIDS, Volume Two: Collected Wisdom.* New York, PWA Coalition, 1988.

Callen, M: *Surviving and Thriving with AIDS, Volume One: Hints for the Newly Diagnosed.* New York, PWA Coalition, 1987.

Glaser, E, and Palmer, L: *In the Absence of Angels.* New York, G.P. Putnam's Sons, 1991. The story of the Glaser family's life with HIV and of Elizabeth Glaser's struggle to get children with HIV included in treatment research.

Kirp, D: *Learning by Heart: AIDS and Schoolchildren in America's Communities.* New Brunswick, New Jersey, Rutgers University Press, 1989.

Kübler-Ross, E: *On Children and Death.* New York, Macmillan Publishing Company, 1985. This book was written especially for parents of children with potentially fatal illnesses. See also, by the same author: *AIDS, the Ultimate Challenge.* New York, Macmillan Publishing Company, 1987.

Kushner, HS: *When Bad Things Happen to Good People.* New York, Avon Books, 1981. Rabbi Kushner's young son died after a long, rare illness. This is his attempt to understand what happened to his family.

Los Angeles Pediatric AIDS Network (LAPAN): *HIV Infection in Children: A Guide for Families.* Los Angeles, LAPAN, 1991. To obtain a copy of the book send $10 to LAPAN, c/o Children's Hospital of Los Angeles, 4650 Sunset Blvd., Box 55, Los Angeles, CA 90027.

McCarroll, T: *Morning Glory Babies.* New York, St. Martin's Press, 1988. The Starcross Community cares for HIV positive children on their farm in Northern California. This is their story.

Oyler, C, with Becklund, L, and Polson, B: *Go Toward the Light.* New York, Harper and Row, 1988. The story of the Oyler family's life when their little son, Ben, got AIDS.

Pizzo, PA, and Wilfert, CM: *Pediatric AIDS: The Challenge of HIV Infection in Infants, Children, and Adolescents.* Baltimore, Williams and Wilkins, 1991. This book is a medical textbook, the first comprehensive one on pediatric HIV infection. Encourage your hospital library to buy a copy, as these books are often quite expensive and this way the information within it can be shared by many readers.

Reider, I, and Ruppelt, P: *AIDS: The Women.* Pittsburgh and San Francisco, Cleis Press, 1988. This book explores the many ways that HIV is affecting the lives of women.

Sherman, M: *Feeding the Sick Child.* Originally written for families with leukemic children, this book is helpful for any parent or caretaker who is having trouble getting their ill child to eat. Write to: Office of Cancer Communications, National Cancer Institute, Bethesda, MD 20014.

Shilts, R: *And the Band Played On. Politics, People and the AIDS Epidemic.* New York, St. Martin's Press, 1987. The history of the AIDS epidemic from 1981-1985. Tough going.

Simon, R: *After the Tears.* Denver, The Children's Museum of Denver, Inc., 1985. Parents talk about raising a child with a disability.

Simonton, OC, Mathews-Simonton, S, and Creighton, J: *Getting Well Again.* Los Angeles, J.P. Tarcher, Inc., 1978. A book about the relationships between life stresses, cancer and immunity, including techniques such as visual imagery for dealing with these stresses and possibly enhancing recovery. Written for adults, the techniques can be taught to children.

Watson, JD: *The Double Helix.* New York, The New American Library, Inc., 1968. The story of the discovery of DNA by one of the two men who did the original work. It tells of Nobel Prizes, professional jealousy, famous scientific personalities and tremendous dedication to an idea. This book is a classic.

In addition to these books, your bookstore, community library and hospital library will have many other books about HIV. One of them, *You Can Do Something About AIDS,* is free. Another is my own *You and Leukemia,* which may be helpful if your child develops an HIV-related cancer.

Also, various national organizations, such as the National Institutes of Health, the Association for the Care of Children's Health (ACCH), the Pediatric AIDS Foundation (PAF), and The Foundation for Children With AIDS; and local organizations such as AIDS Project Los Angeles (APLA), the Gay Men's Health Crisis (GMHC) in New York City, and AIDS Children Teaching Us About Love (ACTUAL) in Brooklyn, publish newsletters, pamphlets and other informational materials. Some of these organizations, and others like them, also provide other services—and most can always use a helping hand. Getting involved with these helping organizations is one more way you can help your child, as well as yourself.

There are two groups of books that I haven't listed but want to mention. One is the group of books written for or about adults with HIV. I included a few of those here because they were recommended to me by parents. Those of you parents who are HIV positive yourselves may want to seek some of these books out as they address more things that grownups worry about than this book could.

Likewise, because this book is for children, it does not discuss the problems of drug abuse or addiction. There are many excellent books available on this subject, and on the kinds of problems families can have as a result. Many children have been exposed to HIV because of a parent's drug abuse, so it is reasonable to assume that some of you are now using drugs, or have in the past. The best places to start looking for information on this subject are AA (Alcoholics Anonymous), Al-Anon and other Twelve-Step programs that exist in all communities. If your family is suffering from these problems in addition to HIV, I strongly encourage you to seek these organizations out. They offer not only information, but support and help.

GLOSSARY OF WORDS NOT DEFINED IN THE TEXT

antacid (ant-*ass'*-ihd)	Medicines that are used to calm down burny-feeling tummys. They come as liquids or as big pills that you suck on until they're gone.
approved medication	A medicine that has been found by the Food and Drug Administration to be both safe and effective when used to treat a certain condition.
arthritis (are-*thry'*-tiss)	Red, hot, swollen, painful joints. Can be caused by many different things.
blood pressure	The force caused by your blood pushing against the walls of your blood vessels.
cephalosporins (seff-ah-low-*spore'*-ins)	One group of antibiotic medicines.
chemicals (*kehm'*-ick-calls)	The stuff that everything is made of, including you.
clotting factors	Proteins in plasma that help your platelets stop blood vessels from leaking and plug them up when you get a cut. Also, a blood product used to treat hemophilia.
experiments (ex-*spare'*-ih-ments)	One of the ways people learn new things. They get an idea of how something might work, and then they figure out how they could prove it, and then try it out to see if it works.
fever	Our bodies are supposed to keep a constant temperature of 98.6 degrees Farenheit. A fever is when your body's temperature gets higher than that.
hemoglobin (*he'*-mow-glow-bin)	The stuff in red blood cells that gives them both their red color and their ability to carry oxygen.
hemophilia (he-mow-*feel'*-ya)	A group of inherited diseases in which a clotting factor isn't made, so people with hemophilia can have trouble bleeding too much or too easily.

latex	A kind of man-made rubber.
molecules (*mah'*-lek-kyoolz)	A very small bit of matter, made up of even smaller things called atoms. Both molecules and atoms are chemicals.
mycobacteria (*my'*-koh-back-*tear'*-ya)	A group of bacteria that are smaller than most others and don't have the same kind of walls. They cause diseases like tuberculosis and leprosy—and MAI.
National Institutes of Health	The most important U.S. government medical research institutions. The two institutes most involved with HIV research are the National Institute of Allergies and Infectious Diseases (NIAID) and the National Cancer Institute (NCI).
operation (opp-er-*ray'*-shun)	A medical procedure done by a surgeon in an operating room.
operating room	A room in a hospital or surgery center where nothing but operations are done. They are kept extremely clean, and are full of shiny equipment, bright lights, and people wearing funny-looking outfits.
pancreatitis (pan-kree-ah-*tie'*-tiss)	A sickness of the pancreas, which is one of your body's factories.
Peds. I.C.U.	Short for Pediatric Intensive Care Unit, these are special wards in hospitals that are set up to take care of either very sick children or children who have just had big operations. They have more nurses and technicians on them than regular wards do.
penicillin (pen-ih-*sill'*-in)	One of the first antibiotics. Both ampicillin and amoxicillin are just newer, improved penicillins that are more useful against certain bacteria.
prescription	A note a doctor writes to a pharmacist telling him or her what medicine to give you. You usually can't read them, and sometimes I wonder how pharmacists can!
procedure (pro-*seed'*-jer)	Just about anything doctors, nurses or technicians do that is more complicated than talking, listening, or taking your pulse, temperature and blood pressure.

protein
(*pro'*-teen)
A special kind of molecule. We are made of proteins, and they do many important jobs in our bodies.

ribs
The ring-like bones around your chest.

sedative
(*said'*-ah-tihv)
A medicine that makes the person who takes it feel very sleepy.

spleen
A large organ that is in the top of the belly on the left side of the body. It does things to keep blood working right and can get very big in certain diseases.

tuberculosis
(too-berk-you-*low'*-siss)
A disease caused by a mycobacterium. It is becoming a common problem for many adults with HIV, but is less common in children. It can be cured with antibiotics.

urine
(*yur'*-in)
The yellow liquid that comes out of your body when you pee. It is made by your kidneys and stored in your bladder until it's time for it to come out.

INDEX